Ellyn Kaschak, PhD
Editor

Minding the Body: Psychotherapy in Cases of Chronic and Life-Threatening Illness

Minding the Body: Psychotherapy in Cases of Chronic and Life-Threatening Illness has been co-published simultaneously as *Women & Therapy,* Volume 23, Number 1 2001.

Pre-publication
REVIEWS,
COMMENTARIES,
EVALUATIONS . . .

"**S**tarting with editor Ellyn Kaschak's impassioned introduction, this collection is AN ENGAGING MIX OF CONTRIBUTIONS THAT OFFER FACTS, COMPELLING FIRST-PERSON ACCOUNTS, AND THEORETICAL/POLITICAL ANALYSIS of chronic illness and the medical business that often disempowers women as it attempts to 'help' them."

Ellen B. Kimmel, PhD
Distinguished Professor
University of South Florida, Tampa

Minding the Body: Psychotherapy in Cases of Chronic and Life-Threatening Illness

Minding the Body: Psychotherapy in Cases of Chronic and Life-Threatening Illness has been co-published simultaneously as *Women & Therapy,* Volume 23, Number 1 2001.

The *Women & Therapy* Monographic "Separates"

Below is a list of "separates," which in serials librarianship means a special issue simultaneously published as a special journal issue or double-issue *and* as a "separate" hardbound monograph. (This is a format which we also call a "DocuSerial.")

"Separates" are published because specialized libraries or professionals may wish to purchase a specific thematic issue by itself in a format which can be separately cataloged and shelved, as opposed to purchasing the journal on an on-going basis. Faculty members may also more easily consider a "separate" for classroom adoption.

"Separates" are carefully classified separately with the major book jobbers so that the journal tie-in can be noted on new book order slips to avoid duplicate purchasing.

You may wish to visit Haworth's website at . . .

http://www.HaworthPress.com

. . . to search our online catalog for complete tables of contents of these separates and related publications.

You may also call 1-800-HAWORTH (outside US/Canada: 607-722-5857), or Fax: 1-800-895-0582 (outside US/Canada: 607-771-0012), or e-mail at:

getinfo@haworthpressinc.com

Minding the Body: Psychotherapy in Cases of Chronic and Life-Threatening Illness, edited by Ellyn Kaschak, PhD (Vol. 23, No. 1, 2001). *Being diagnosed with cancer, lupus, or fibromyalgia is a traumatic event. All too often, women are told their disease is 'all in their heads' and therefore both 'unreal and insignificant' by a medical profession that dismisses emotions and scorns mental illness. Combining personal narratives and theoretical views of illness, Minding the Body offers an alternative approach to the mind-body connection. This book shows the reader how to deal with the painful and difficult emotions that exacerbate illness, while learning the emotional and spiritual lessons illness can teach.*

For Love or Money: The Fee in Feminist Therapy, edited by Marcia Hill, EdD, and Ellyn Kaschak, PhD (Vol. 22, No. 3, 1999). *"Recommended reading for both new and seasoned professionals . . . . An exciting and timely book about 'the last taboo' . . . . " (Carolyn C. Larsen, PhD, Senior Counsellor Emeritus, University of Calgary; Partner, Alberta Psychological Resources Ltd., Calgary, and Co-editor, Ethical Decision Making in Therapy: Feminist Perspectives)*

Beyond the Rule Book: Moral Issues and Dilemmas in the Practice of Psychotherapy, edited by Ellyn Kaschak, PhD, and Marcia Hill, EdD (Vol. 22, No. 2, 1999). *"The authors in this important and timely book tackle the difficult task of working through . . . conflicts, sharing their moral struggles and real life solutions in working with diverse populations and in a variety of clinical settings. . . . Will provide psychotherapists with a thought-provoking source for the stimulating and essential discussion of our own and our profession's moral bases." (Carolyn C. Larsen, PhD, Senior Counsellor Emeritus, University of Calgary, Partner in private practice, Alberta Psychological Resources Ltd., Calgary, and Co-editor, Ethical Decision Making in Therapy: Feminist Perspectives)*

Assault on the Soul: Women in the Former Yugoslavia, edited by Sara Sharratt, PhD, and Ellyn Kaschak, PhD (Vol. 22, No. 1, 1999). *Explores the applications and intersections of feminist therapy, activism and jurisprudence with women and children in the former Yugoslavia.*

Learning from Our Mistakes: Difficulties and Failures in Feminist Therapy, edited by Marcia Hill, EdD, and Esther D. Rothblum, PhD (Vol. 21, No. 3, 1998). *"A courageous and fundamental step in evolving a well-grounded body of theory and of investigating the assumptions that unexamined, lead us to error." (Teresa Bernardez, MD, Training and Supervising Analyst, The Michigan Psychoanalytic Council)*

Feminist Therapy as a Political Act, edited by Marcia Hill, EdD (Vol. 21, No. 2, 1998). *"A real contribution to the field. . . . A valuable tool for feminist therapists and those who want to learn about feminist therapy." (Florence L. Denmark, PhD, Robert S. Pace Distinguished Professor of Psychology and Chair, Psychology Department, Pace University, New York, New York)*

Breaking the Rules: Women in Prison and Feminist Therapy, edited by Judy Harden, PhD, and Marcia Hill, EdD (Vol. 20, No. 4 & Vol. 21, No. 1, 1998). *"Fills a long-recognized gap in the psychology of women curricula, demonstrating that feminist theory can be made relevant to the practice of feminism, even in prison." (Suzanne J. Kessler, PhD, Professor of Psychology and Women's Studies, State University of New York at Purchase)*

Children's Rights, Therapists' Responsibilities: Feminist Commentaries, edited by Gail Anderson, MA, and Marcia Hill, EdD (Vol. 20, No. 2, 1997). *"Addresses specific practice dimensions that will help therapists organize and resolve conflicts about working with children, adolescents, and their families in therapy." (Feminist Bookstore News)*

More than a Mirror: How Clients Influence Therapists' Lives, edited by Marcia Hill, EdD (Vol. 20, No. 1, 1997). *"Courageous, insightful, and deeply moving. These pages reveal the scrupulous self-examination and self-reflection of conscientious therapists at their best. AN IMPORTANT CONTRIBUTION TO FEMINIST THERAPY LITERATURE AND A BOOK WORTH READING BY THERAPISTS AND CLIENTS ALIKE." (Rachel Josefowitz Siegal, MSW, retired feminist therapy practitioner; Co-Editor, Women Changing Therapy; Jewish Women in Therapy; and Celebrating the Lives of Jewish Women: Patterns in a Feminist Sampler)*

Sexualities, edited by Marny Hall, PhD, LCSW (Vol. 19, No. 4, 1997). *"Explores the diverse and multifaceted nature of female sexuality, covering topics including sadomasochism in the therapy room, sexual exploitation in cults, and genderbending in cyberspace." (Feminist Bookstore News)*

Couples Therapy: Feminist Perspectives, edited by Marcia Hill, EdD, and Esther D. Rothblum, PhD (Vol. 19, No. 3, 1996). *Addresses some of the inadequacies, omissions, and assumptions in traditional couples' therapy to help you face the issues of race, ethnicity, and sexual orientation in helping couples today.*

A Feminist Clinician's Guide to the Memory Debate, edited by Susan Contratto, PhD, and M. Janice Gutfreund, PhD (Vol. 19, No. 1, 1996). *"Unites diverse scholars, clinicians, and activists in an insightful and useful examination of the issues related to recovered memories." (Feminist Bookstore News)*

Classism and Feminist Therapy: Counting Costs, edited by Marcia Hill, EdD, and Esther D. Rothblum, PhD (Vol. 18, No. 3/4, 1996). *"EDUCATES, CHALLENGES, AND QUESTIONS THE INFLUENCE OF CLASSISM ON THE CLINICAL PRACTICE OF PSYCHOTHERAPY WITH WOMEN." (Kathleen P. Gates, MA, Certified Professional Counselor, Center for Psychological Health, Superior, Wisconsin)*

Lesbian Therapists and Their Therapy: From Both Sides of the Couch, edited by Nancy D. Davis, MD, Ellen Cole, PhD, and Esther D. Rothblum, PhD (Vol. 18, No. 2, 1996). *"Highlights the power and boundary issues of psychotherapy from perspectives that many readers may have neither considered nor experienced in their own professional lives." (Psychiatric Services)*

Feminist Foremothers in Women's Studies, Psychology, and Mental Health, edited by Phyllis Chesler, PhD, Esther D. Rothblum, PhD, and Ellen Cole, PhD (Vol. 17, No. 1/2/3/4, 1995). *"A must for feminist scholars and teachers . . . These women's personal experiences are poignant and powerful." (Women's Studies International Forum)*

Women's Spirituality, Women's Lives, edited by Judith Ochshorn, PhD, and Ellen Cole, PhD (Vol. 16, No. 2/3, 1995). *"A delightful and complex book on spirituality and sacredness in women's lives." (Joan Clingan, MA, Spiritual Psychology, Graduate Advisor, Prescott College Master of Arts Program)*

Psychopharmacology from a Feminist Perspective, edited by Jean A. Hamilton, MD, Margaret Jensvold, MD, Esther D. Rothblum, PhD, and Ellen Cole, PhD (Vol. 16, No. 1, 1995). *"Challenges readers to increase* *their sensitivity and awareness of the role of sex and gender in response to and acceptance of pharmacologic therapy."* (American Journal of Pharmaceutical Education)

Wilderness Therapy for Women: The Power of Adventure, edited by Ellen Cole, PhD, Esther D. Rothblum, PhD, and Eve Erdman, MEd, MLS (Vol. 15, No. 3/4, 1994). *"There's an undeniable excitement in these pages about the thrilling satisfaction of meeting challenges in the physical world, the world outside our cities that is unfamiliar, uneasy territory for many women. If you're interested at all in the subject, this book is well worth your time."* (Psychology of Women Quarterly)

Bringing Ethics Alive: Feminist Ethics in Psychotherapy Practice, edited by Nanette K. Gartrell, MD (Vol. 15, No. 1, 1994). *"Examines the theoretical and practical issues of ethics in feminist therapies. From the responsibilities of training programs to include social issues ranging from racism to sexism to practice ethics, this outlines real questions and concerns."* (Midwest Book Review)

Women with Disabilities: Found Voices, edited by Mary Willmuth, PhD, and Lillian Holcomb, PhD (Vol. 14, No. 3/4, 1994). *"These powerful chapters often jolt the anti-disability consciousness and force readers to contend with the ways in which disability has been constructed, disguised, and rendered disgusting by much of society."* (Academic Library Book Review)

Faces of Women and Aging, edited by Nancy D. Davis, MD, Ellen Cole, PhD, and Esther D. Rothblum, PhD (Vol. 14, No. 1/2, 1993). *"This uplifting, helpful book is of great value not only for aging women, but also for women of all ages who are interested in taking active control of their own lives."* (New Mature Woman)

Refugee Women and Their Mental Health: Shattered Societies, Shattered Lives, edited by Ellen Cole, PhD, Oliva M. Espin, PhD, and Esther D. Rothblum, PhD (Vol. 13, No. 1/2/3, 1992). *"The ideas presented are rich and the perspectives varied, and the book is an important contribution to understanding refugee women in a global context."* (Comtemporary Psychology)

Women, Girls and Psychotherapy: Reframing Resistance, edited by Carol Gilligan, PhD, Annie Rogers, PhD, and Deborah Tolman, EdD (Vol. 11, No. 3/4, 1991). *"Of use to educators, psychotherapists, and parents–in short, to any person who is directly involved with girls at adolescence."* (Harvard Educational Review)

Professional Training for Feminist Therapists: Personal Memoirs, edited by Esther D. Rothblum, PhD, and Ellen Cole, PhD (Vol. 11, No. 1, 1991). *"Exciting, interesting, and filled with the angst and the energies that directed these women to develop an entirely different approach to counseling."* (Science Books & Films)

Jewish Women in Therapy: Seen But Not Heard, edited by Rachel Josefowitz Siegel, MSW, and Ellen Cole, PhD (Vol. 10, No. 4, 1991). *"A varied collection of prose and poetry, first-person stories, and accessible theoretical pieces that can help Jews and non-Jews, women and men, therapists and patients, and general readers to grapple with questions of Jewish women's identities and diversity."* (Canadian Psychology)

Women's Mental Health in Africa, edited by Esther D. Rothblum, PhD, and Ellen Cole, PhD (Vol. 10, No. 3, 1990). *"A valuable contribution and will be of particular interest to scholars in women's studies, mental health, and cross-cultural psychology."* (Contemporary Psychology)

Motherhood: A Feminist Perspective, edited by Jane Price Knowles, MD, and Ellen Cole, PhD (Vol. 10, No. 1/2, 1990). *"Provides some enlightening perspectives. . . . It is worth the time of both male and female readers."* (Comtemporary Psychology)

Diversity and Complexity in Feminist Therapy, edited by Laura Brown, PhD, ABPP, and Maria P. P. Root, PhD (Vol. 9, No. 1/2, 1990). *"A most convincing discussion and illustration of the importance of adopting a multicultural perspective for theory building in feminist therapy. . . . THIS BOOK IS A MUST FOR THERAPISTS and should be included on psychology of women syllabi."* (Association for Women in Psychology Newsletter)

Fat Opression and Psychotherapy, edited by Laura S. Brown, PhD, and Esther D. Rothblum, PhD (Vol. 8, No. 3, 1990). *"Challenges many traditional beliefs about being fat . . . A refreshing new* *perspective for approaching and thinking about issues related to weight.'' (Association for Women in Psychology Newsletter)*

Lesbianism: Affirming Nontraditional Roles, edited by Esther D. Rothblum, PhD, and Ellen Cole, PhD (Vol. 8, No. 1/2, 1989). *"Touches on many of the most significant issues brought before therapists today." (Newsletter of the Association of Gay & Lesbian Psychiatrists)*

Women and Sex Therapy: Closing the Circle of Sexual Knowledge, edited by Ellen Cole, PhD, and Esther D. Rothblum, PhD (Vol. 7, No. 2/3, 1989). *"ADDS IMMEASUREABLY TO THE FEMINIST THERAPY LITERATURE THAT DISPELS MALE PARADIGMS OF PATHOLOGY WITH REGARD TO WOMEN." (Journal of Sex Education & Therapy)*

The Politics of Race and Gender in Therapy, edited by Lenora Fulani, PhD (Vol. 6, No. 4, 1988). *Women of color examine newer therapies that encourage them to develop their historical identity.*

Treating Women's Fear of Failure, edited by Esther D. Rothblum, PhD, and Ellen Cole, PhD (Vol. 6, No. 3, 1988). *"SHOULD BE RECOMMENDED READING FOR ALL MENTAL HEALTH PROFESSIONALS, SOCIAL WORKERS, EDUCATORS, AND VOCATIONAL COUNSELORS WHO WORK WITH WOMEN." (The Journal of Clinical Psychiatry)*

Women, Power, and Therapy: Issues for Women, edited by Marjorie Braude, MD (Vol. 6, No. 1/2, 1987). *"RAISE[S] THERAPISTS' CONSCIOUSNESS ABOUT THE IMPORTANCE OF CONSIDERING GENDER-BASED POWER IN THERAPY. . . welcome contribution.'' (Australian Journal of Psychology)*

Dynamics of Feminist Therapy, edited by Doris Howard (Vol. 5, No. 2/3, 1987). *"A comprehensive treatment of an important and vexing subject.'' (Australian Journal of Sex, Marriage and Family)*

A Woman's Recovery from the Trauma of War: Twelve Responses from Feminist Therapists and Activists, edited by Esther D. Rothblum, PhD, and Ellen Cole, PhD (Vol. 5, No. 1, 1986). *"A MILESTONE. In it, twelve women pay very close attention to a woman who has been deeply wounded by war." (The World)*

Women and Mental Health: New Directions for Change, edited by Carol T. Mowbray, PhD, Susan Lanir, MA, and Marilyn Hulce, MSW, ACSW (Vol. 3, No. 3/4, 1985). *"The overview of sex differences in disorders is clear and sensitive, as is the review of sexual exploitation of clients by therapists. . . . MANDATORY READING FOR ALL THERAPISTS WHO WORK WITH WOMEN." (British Journal of Medical Psychology and The British Psychological Society)*

Women Changing Therapy: New Assessments, Values, and Strategies in Feminist Therapy, edited by Joan Hamerman Robbins and Rachel Josefowitz Siegel, MSW (Vol. 2, No. 2/3, 1983). *"An excellent collection to use in teaching therapists that reflection and resolution in treatment do not simply lead tp adaptation, but to an active inner process of judging.'' (News for Women in Psychiatry)*

Current Feminist Issues in Psychotherapy, edited by The New England Association for Women in Psychology (Vol. 1, No. 3, 1983). *Addresses depression, displaced homemakers, sibling incest, and body image from a feminist perspective.*

Minding the Body: Psychotherapy in Cases of Chronic and Life-Threatening Illness

Ellyn Kaschak, PhD
Editor

Minding the Body: Psychotherapy in Cases of Chronic and Life-Threatening Illness has been co-published simultaneously as *Women & Therapy,* Volume 23, Number 1 2001.

The Haworth Press, Inc.
New York • London • Oxford

Minding the Body: Psychotherapy in Cases of Chronic and Life-Threatening Illness has been co-published simultaneously as *Women & Therapy* ™, Volume 23, Number 1 2001.

The development, preparation, and publication of this work has been undertaken with great care. However, the publisher, employees, editors, and agents of The Haworth Press and all imprints of The Haworth Press, Inc., including The Haworth Medical Press® and Pharmaceutical Products Press®, are not responsible for any errors contained herein or for consequences that may ensue from use of materials or information contained in this work. Opinions expressed by the author(s) are not necessarily those of The Haworth Press, Inc.

The Haworth Press, Inc., 10 Alice Street, Binghamton, NY 13904-1580 USA

Cover design by Jennifer M. Gaska

Library of Congress Cataloging-in-Publication Data

Minding the body : psychotherapy in cases of chronic and life-threatening illness / Ellyn Kaschak, editor.
     p. cm.
    Includes bibliographical references and index.
    ISBN 0-7890-1367-3 (hard : alk. paper)–ISBN 0-7890-1368-1 (pbk : alk. paper)
     1. Feminist therapy. 2. Women analysands–Health and hygiene. 3. Chronically ill–Care. 4. Critically ill–Care. I. Kaschak, Ellyn, 1943-
     [DNLM: 1. Chronic Disease–psychology. 2. Critical Illness–psychology. 3. Neoplasms–psychology. 4. Psychotherapy. 5. Women–psychology. WT 500 M663 2001]
    RC489.F45 M54 2001
    616.89′14′082–dc21
                                                    00-054706

Indexing, Abstracting & Website/Internet Coverage

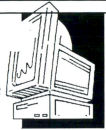

   This section provides you with a list of major indexing & abstracting services. That is to say, each service began covering this periodical during the year noted in the right column. Most Websites which are listed below have indicated that they will either post, disseminate, compile, archive, cite or alert their own Website users with research-based content from this work. (This list is as current as the copyright date of this publication.)

Abstracting, Website/Indexing Coverage .... Year When Coverage Began

- *Academic Abstracts/CD-ROM* **1995**
- *Academic Index (on-line)* **1992**
- *Academic Search Elite (EBSCO)* **1994**
- *Alternative Press Index (online & CD-ROM from NISC)*
  <www.nisc.com> **1982**
- *Behavioral Medicine Abstracts* **1996**
- *BUBL Information Service, an Internet-based Information*
  Service for the UK higher education community
  <URL: http://bubl.ac.uk/> **1995**
- *Child Development & Bibliography (in print & online)* **1994**
- *CNPIEC Reference Guide: Chinese National Directory*
  of Foreign Periodicals **1996**
- *Contemporary Women's Issues* **1998**
- *Current Contents: Social & Behavioral Sciences*
  <www.isinet.com> **1995**
- *Expanded Academic Index* **1993**
- *Family Studies Database (online and CD/ROM)*
  <www.nisc.com> **1996**

(continued)

(continued)

Special Bibliographic Notes related to special journal issues (separates) and indexing/abstracting:

- indexing/abstracting services in this list will also cover material in any "separate" that is co-published simultaneously with Haworth's special thematic journal issue or DocuSerial. Indexing/abstracting usually covers material at the article/chapter level.
- monographic co-editions are intended for either non-subscribers or libraries which intend to purchase a second copy for their circulating collections.
- monographic co-editions are reported to all jobbers/wholesalers/approval plans. The source journal is listed as the "series" to assist the prevention of duplicate purchasing in the same manner utilized for books-in-series.
- to facilitate user/access services all indexing/abstracting services are encouraged to utilize the co-indexing entry note indicated at the bottom of the first page of each article/chapter/contribution.
- this is intended to assist a library user of any reference tool (whether print, electronic, online, or CD-ROM) to locate the monographic version if the library has purchased this version but not a subscription to the source journal.
- individual articles/chapters in any Haworth publication are also available through the Haworth Document Delivery Service (HDDS).

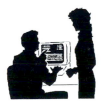

ABOUT THE EDITOR

Ellyn Kaschak, PhD, is Professor of Psychology at San Jose State University in San Jose, California. She is author of *Engendered Lives: A New Psychology of Women's Experience*, as well as numerous articles and chapters on feminist psychology and psychotherapy. Dr. Kaschak is also co-editor of *Assault on the Soul: Women in the Former Yugoslavia*, *Beyond the Rule Book: Moral Issues and Dilemmas in the Practice of Psychotherapy* and *For Love or Money: The Fee in Feminist Therapy*. She has had thirty years of experience practicing psychotherapy, is past Chair of the Feminist Therapy Institute and of the APA Committee on Women and is Fellow of Division 35, the Psychology of Women, Division 12, Clinical Psychology, Division 45, Ethnic Minority Issues and Division 52, International Psychology, of the American Psychological Association. She is co-editor of the journal *Women & Therapy*.

Minding the Body: Psychotherapy in Cases of Chronic and Life-Threatening Illness

CONTENTS

This volume is dedicated to all the women who did not have time enough to tell their stories.

Minding the Body:
Psychotherapy in Cases of Chronic
and Life-Threatening Illness

Ellyn Kaschak

I did not choose this topic. Rather it chose me. Would I have developed an interest in chronic and life-threatening illness had it not sought me out? I do not know. Perhaps I would have had the impulse to turn away in a self-protective gesture or to read about it only if and when I was faced with a client whose case demanded such knowledge. As is so for many of us who do not have the luxury of choice, the privilege not to deal with sexism, racism, anti-Semitism, disability or homophobia, an increasing number of us also have the choice to deal with chronic and life-threatening illness made for us.

When I was growing up, cancer was not talked about, even the word itself was spoken in hushed tones, if at all. That questionable luxury has also been taken from us. Given the startling statistics involving the growing incidence of illnesses such as the many forms of cancer and autoimmune disorders among people in general and women in particular, even more of us will be directly affected by contracting one of these diseases or having someone close to us do so. Those of us who have not yet confronted these issues with clients soon will. In the United States, one in three individuals will have some form of cancer in their lifetime. The number of individuals diagnosed with the various autoimmune disorders is steadily increasing and women are differentially impacted. Women are more frequently diagnosed with these illnesses in varying ratios depending upon the specific malady (Chrisler, this volume). This does not include those who go undiagnosed or misdiagnosed.

As therapists we have much to learn and much to contribute to the understanding and treatment of these disorders. We must question society's and the

[Haworth co-indexing entry note]: "Minding the Body: Psychotherapy in Cases of Chronic and Life-Threatening Illness." Kaschak, Ellyn. Co-published simultaneously in *Women & Therapy* (The Haworth Press, Inc.) Vol. 23, No. 1, 2001, pp. 1-5; and: *Minding the Body: Psychotherapy in Cases of Chronic and Life-Threatening Illness* (ed: Ellyn Kaschak) The Haworth Press, Inc., 2001, pp. 1-5. Single or multiple copies of this article are available for a fee from The Haworth Document Delivery Service [1-800-342-9678, 9:00 a.m. - 5:00 p.m. (EST). E-mail address: getinfo@haworthpressinc.com].

1

medical profession's constructs and concepts about these illnesses, as well as the treatment of each woman involved. As feminists, we bring to bear a healthy skepticism about traditional concepts and treatment methods in general and in particular when women are the focus. And sadly we are not disappointed.

We all live on the same poisoned planet and none of us and none of our clients are more than temporarily safe from harm. One can try to maintain the separateness that is so endemic to Western thought and Western life, think only of oneself or one's immediate intimates. Yet it is apparent to feminists that such divided and divisive concepts are false, that they are defied even by our own bodies. The poisons that are so clearly implicated in these illnesses are in all of our bodies, those already diagnosed and those as yet undiagnosed.

Chemicals in the air, the water, the ground and the food supply are being acknowledged as more causatively significant than genetic anomalies for cancer. The pesticides in our food and water were originally developed for use in warfare in World War II and are now used against ourselves and against all of humanity. In a form of massive self-destruction, we have all become the enemy and are killing ourselves. Yet, as with so many other inventions of modern science, they are no longer intended to kill anyone. Nor are they intended not to. In the illusory boundaries constructed by modern science and modern pharmacology, these are only "side effects." And in yet another stroke of epistemological and economic chicanery, the same corporate structure that produces the poisons which are wounding and killing us by the millions has created a ready market for the curative poisons, the chemotherapy and radiation.

More recently genetic engineering of food has been added to the scientific armamentarium and to the corporate ledger with virtually no knowledge of what these monstrous mixtures create within each human body, each cell. By the time this question is answered, it will be too late. Just as science is beginning to learn about the complex and multiple aspects of the immune system and the genetic code, it is also complicit in their violation, if not destruction.

There is yet another distinction that continues both culturally and professionally despite demonstration after demonstration to the contrary and that is the Cartesian notion of the separation of mind and body. Medical professionals who are willing to consider the separate sphere of mind as at least influencing the physical are considered progressive. This is nineteenth century epistemology. That each is embedded in the other, that mind is everywhere and not just in the brain is yet to be accepted by much of 21st century medicine.

Just as important is the philosophical materialism that continues to pervade the medical professions in Western society, culminating in a disrespect for psychology, a view of the mind as a trickster and the material as reality. Nowhere is it more evident than in discussions of the much maligned placebo effect, which is rarely taken seriously enough to be investigated and understood by science. Instead this well-known phenomenon is typically taken as a prima facia demonstration that a patient has been tricked by methodology, by a modern form of hysteria. Because the cure comes from the mind rather than the medicine, it is considered a cure that is not a cure, but rather a demonstration that there never was an illness at all. It becomes an embarrassment to be cured of something by this route. By this solipsistic reasoning, such a remission is taken as proof that something was actually nothing.

This prejudice is manifested differently in relation to the two major categories of illness considered here. For autoimmune diseases, the question of the medical profession has been, "Is it real or psychological?" This is entirely the wrong question, one based not only in a dualistic epistemology, but even more deeply in a bias against "women's illnesses." How long will the concept of hysteria continue to be dressed in contemporary garb and used to demean women's real problems?

With regard to cancer, prolonging life as a result of psychotherapy or participation in a support group is typically not viewed as valid and "real" as from physical medicine, particularly the harshest forms such as chemotherapy. The early and continuing psychological interventions of Lawrence LeShan (1989) with terminal cancer patients have produced a better rate of remission with certain patients than any known form of chemotherapy. David Spiegel (1989) also demonstrated that the lives of women with terminal breast cancer were extended for a mean of eighteen months beyond those of controls by participation in support groups. Not only do these results defy the separation of mind and body, but they underline a crucial role for psychology and psychiatry in the treatment of these illnesses.

These are the largest issues, the theoretical and political. In the practice of feminist psychotherapy the largest vista is context for the most intimate terrain. The therapy relationship must be spacious, allowing room for political outrage and tender support, revolutionary theory and loving intimacy, all organized by the personal meanings and multiple effects that any illness has on an individual life, on a relationship, a family and a community. What happens to a woman, to her life, when she hears one of these diagnoses, when she survives not just one of these illnesses, but the treatments of it and the treatment of her by the medical profession? To a woman who hears that she has no diagnosis, that it is all "in her head," a less valid location than in her body? After all, we do not have any such dismissive expression as "It's all in your body."

The tasks of the psychotherapist working in these circumstances are diverse and multiple. Many of them are already well known to us; some require innovation. As with many of the traumas in women's lives, psychotherapists are often called upon after the fact, after the injury or illness has taken its toll. In these cases, we know how to deal with fear and grief, loss and disappointment, the shame and self-blame that can be experienced in such circumstances. We already have expertise in dealing with questions of identity that arise, with the question, "Am I the same person that I was before this diagnosis?" We know how to offer support and encouragement while allowing any experience and every truth to be voiced. We know how to offer appreciation for women's strength, resilience and courage.

It is often a complete surprise to the patient herself to see who stands by her and who turns away at such a time. A circumstance of grave illness unfortunately can become a test of friendship and love, courage and integrity. Women are too often the designated caretakers in relationships and receive support and care in circumstances of their own illness less frequently than do men. More often than not, their caretaking obligations and concerns continue even in times of great peril to themselves.

For the therapist who has not experienced these illnesses herself, it can be surprising to begin to perceive that such life crises are also very often fertile ground for deep experiences of personal transformation and spiritual awakening. For the family and friends who are able to provide support and love, the deepening of bonds and relationships can be unparalleled.

Feminist therapy must also be engaged in prevention of the circumstances that are implicated in the growing epidemics of these illnesses. These include theoretically an epistemology that disconnects cause and effect, body and mind, materially a poisoned planet and psychologically the intense stress and trauma in many contemporary women's lives that, if left untreated, can result in the breakdown of the immune system.

Finally, with whatever influence we have, whatever voices we can raise, we must continue to demand the integration of the professions that deal with different aspects of illness, of human functioning as if they were indeed separate. We must work toward a complex, contextual and holistic concept of people and an appropriate professional integration of practices that treat human illness, such as psychotherapy, acupuncture, herbal medicine, Eastern practices, Western medicine, nutrition, spiritual practices and other approaches amply demonstrated to impact health and illness alike.

The articles dealing with these illnesses range from the intimate to the academic, the personal to the scholarly, that admixture that is the hallmark of feminist psychology. Joan Chrisler presents an overview of issues involved in dealing with women diagnosed with autoimmune disorders, while Mary White, Jeanne Parr Lemkau and Mark Clasen discuss the specifics of fibromyalgia. These articles are complemented by that of Paula Caplan, who describes her struggle to arrive at an accurate diagnosis for Chronic Fatigue Syndrome. Interestingly, Caplan is an expert on psychological diagnoses and issues involving the DSM and found herself embroiled in an analogous situation in seeking an accurate diagnosis of her own illness. Judy Lerner and Maureen Reid-Cunningham present a personal and professional discussion of Lerner's illness (fibromyalgia) and injury (broken leg). The therapist and client together discuss the effects of their mutual experience of illness and the course of therapy based on a feminist relational model.

Suni Petersen and Lois Banishek present an incisive discussion of the social construction of illness, particularly cancer, along with important suggestions for treatment from a social constructivist perspective. This article is followed by personal accounts of dealing with cancer by two psychotherapists. Pamela Fischer cogently describes her own experience with breast cancer and what it taught her about her work. Denise Twohey also writes from the dual perspective of a feminist therapist and a patient who underwent surgery for the removal of a malignant brain tumor. Finally, Juli Burnell discusses her life-threatening brain illness and its effects on her understanding about her own work and her own clients.

All these women who have courageously written about their own experiences have taken an important step in healing their own wounds and in helping others to do so. As feminists, we resist an individualistic and fragmenting culture that conspires to divide us from ourselves and each other. We seek the sources of problems in the culture and not just inside the individual and solutions in healing the divisions and fragmentations between us and within us. We suffer from reductionist science, corporate greed and the frequent hubris of the medical profession as much as we suffer from the personal losses and agonies of having any one of these illnesses visited upon us. We suffer and die from a poisoned environment and fragmenting culture, from contextual illness. For we are not separate from this context and what begins as context ends as self.

REFERENCES

LeShan, Lawrence (1989). Cancer as a Turning Point. E. P. Dutton: New York.
Spiegel, David et al. (1989). A psychosocial intervention and survival time of patients with metastatic breast cancer. *The Lancet*, volume 2, 888-891.

How Can Feminist Therapists Support Women with Autoimmune Disorders?

Joan C. Chrisler

SUMMARY. Although many autoimmune disorders are unfamiliar to most Americans, together these disorders represent a significant proportion of the total incidence of chronic disease. Women are diagnosed with autoimmune disorders more often than men, and the sex difference is substantial in some disorders. The peak age of onset of these disorders is from early adulthood to mid-life, which violates the popular assumption that only older people experience chronic, debilitating illnesses. The unpredictability of autoimmune disorders, the knowledge that they are progressive and incurable, the possibility of deleterious treatment side-effects, and the general public's unfamiliarity with autoimmune disorders combine to make living with one a frustrating and isolating experience. The purposes of this article are to educate feminist therapists about autoimmune disorders and to encourage feminist therapists to use their expertise to help support women who are adjusting to life with an autoimmune disorder. *[Article copies available for a fee from The Haworth Document Delivery Service: 1-800-342-9678. E-mail address: <getinfo@haworthpressinc.com> Website: <http://www.HaworthPress.com> © 2001 by The Haworth Press, Inc. All rights reserved.]*

KEYWORDS. Autoimmune disorders, adaptation to chronic illness, women and chronic illness, rheumatoid arthritis, lupus

Joan C. Chrisler, PhD, is Professor of Psychology at Connecticut College, where she teaches courses on health psychology and the psychology of women.

Address correspondence to: Joan C. Chrisler, PhD, Department of Psychology, Connecticut College, New London, CT 06320 (E-mail: jcchr@conncoll.edu).

[Haworth co-indexing entry note]: "How Can Feminist Therapists Support Women with Autoimmune Disorders?" Chrisler, Joan C. Co-published simultaneously in *Women & Therapy* (The Haworth Press, Inc.) Vol. 23, No. 1, 2001, pp. 7-22; and: *Minding the Body: Psychotherapy in Cases of Chronic and Life-Threatening Illness* (ed: Ellyn Kaschak) The Haworth Press, Inc., 2001, pp. 7-22. Single or multiple copies of this article are available for a fee from The Haworth Document Delivery Service [1-800-342-9678, 9:00 a.m. - 5:00 p.m. (EST). E-mail address: getinfo@haworthpressinc.com].

7

All people with chronic illnesses have one thing in common: they "will never again return to the pre-illness sense of self, of options, of invulnerability, of obliviousness to the body's functioning" (Goodheart & Lansing, 1997, p. 3). They must live with the awareness that they will not get better and that they might get worse (Goodheart & Lansing, 1997). A diagnosis of chronic illness requires people to confront and cope with a set of potential threats. Among the threats noted by Favlo (1991) are threats to life; physical, psychological, and economic well-being; bodily integrity; relationships with family, friends, and colleagues; independence, privacy, autonomy, and control; self-concept; life goals; and ability to meet role obligations. Many studies of people with chronic illness have found anxiety and depression to be widespread among them (Taylor, 1999), and it's no wonder. Coping with symptoms, treatments, and threats; revising one's self-concept; and adjusting one's behavioral routines and role obligations constitute a heavy burden.

Although it may seem obvious that people who have recently been diagnosed with a chronic illness would benefit from the support and guidance of a good psychotherapist, the fact remains that people with chronic diseases are an underserved population (Goodheart & Lansing, 1997). Many physicians and psychotherapists do not understand the need for psychosocial support of people with chronic illnesses. Physicians may not refer their patients for psychotherapy out of ignorance of how it might be helpful, unwillingness to address patients' psychological symptoms and concerns, or a belief that psychotherapy is an alternative, rather than a complementary, treatment (Knight & Camic, 1998). Psychotherapists may not reach out to people with chronic illnesses or to physicians for referrals because they think that their lack of training in medicine or health psychology makes them unfit for the task, because they believe that patients get the support they need from medical personnel, or because of their own anxiety about being around or working with people who have chronic diseases (Goodheart & Lansing, 1997).

Feminist therapists already have the skills necessary to help people with chronic illness cope with anxiety, depression, role changes, stigma, and adjustment. They are particularly able to assist women with gendered illness concerns, such as body image and sexuality changes, reproductive decision making, and relationship complications. Furthermore, feminist therapists may be perceived as a particularly comforting source of support and advice for clients with illnesses, such as autoimmune disorders, that are more common in women. If you have not yet worked with a client with chronic illness and are not particularly interested in physical health, you may be wondering whether you should read on. Someday a new client may present herself to ask you for help in adjusting to a recent diagnosis of lupus or multiple sclerosis, or a current client may mention in the course of a regular session that she has been diagnosed with Grave's disease or Sjogren's syndrome and ask if you know anything about it. I hope you will want to prepare yourself for the challenge and satisfaction of supporting women with chronic illness.

AUTOIMMUNE DISORDERS

Autoimmune disorders result when the immune system fails to discriminate between self and non-self, and thus produces autoantibodies that attack the body's own cells. Autoantibodies may be either specific (e.g., thyroid or blood autoantibodies) and associated with single-organ diseases or non-specific (e.g., antinuclear antibodies) and associated with multi-system diseases (Ollier & Symmons, 1992). Autoantibodies do not necessarily destroy the target tissue; some achieve their effects by deranging the function of the organ or tissue (Crowley, 1997). The reasons why individuals form autoantibodies are not yet clear, but several mechanisms have been postulated. The most likely of these are that (a) the patient's own antigens have been altered by some substance (e.g., drug, virus, environmental toxin) that causes them to become antigenic and provoke autoimmune reactions; (b) cross-reacting antibodies against foreign substances are formed and then also attack the body's own tissues; or (c) the body's regulator T-lymphocytes are defective and misregulate the immune system's responses (Crowley, 1997).

Among the more common of the autoimmune disorders are multiple sclerosis (MS), rheumatoid arthritis (RA), Grave's disease, Hashimoto's thyroiditis, pernicious anemia, type 1 diabetes mellitus, chronic active hepatitis, systemic lupus erythematosus (SLE), Sjogren's syndrome, glomerulonephritis, scleroderma, and myasthenia gravis (Carlson, Eisenstat, & Ziporyn, 1996; Crowley, 1997; Merck Research Laboratories, 1992; Ollier & Symmons, 1992). Chronic fatigue syndrome (CFS), irritable bowel syndrome (IBS), vasculitis, and other chronic disorders of unknown etiology are under investigation for evidence of autoimmunity (Ollier & Symmons, 1992). Together the above disorders represent a significant proportion of the total incidence of chronic disease.

Women are diagnosed with autoimmune disorders more often than men, and in the case of some disorders the sex difference in prevalence is substantial. The female to male ratio of patients with SLE, Sjogren's syndrome, and Hashimoto's thyroiditis is 9:1. The ratio is 6:1 for Grave's disease, 3:1 for RA, chronic active hepatitis, scleroderma, and myasthenia gravis, and 1.5:1 for MS and pernicious anemia (Ollier & Symmons, 1992). The peak age of onset of autoimmune disorders tends to be in mid-life. For example, people tend to be diagnosed with SLE between the ages of 20 to 40, RA 30 to 50, Grave's disease 20 to 40, Hashimoto's thyroiditis 40 to 60, myasthenia gravis 20 to 30, Sjogren's syndrome around age 50, and MS around age 30 (Ollier & Symmons, 1992).

The greater frequency of most autoimmune disorders in women and age distributions that show increased incidence coinciding with periods of marked alterations in endocrine functioning (e.g., pregnancy, perimenopause) have led researchers to suggest that gonadal hormones may be involved (Kiecolt-Glaser & Glaser, 1988). Evidence for the involvement of estrogenic hormones has been noted in women with SLE and RA. Oral contraceptives can exacerbate symptoms of SLE; flare-ups are common during pregnancy and postpartum, and both women and men with disorders that involve excessive estrogen exposure are at increased risk of developing SLE (Achterberg-Lawlis, 1988; Kiecolt-Glaser & Glaser, 1988). RA is rare before puberty, and its incidence is much greater in women than in men during the reproductive years than it is after menopause (Ollier & Symmons, 1992). Furthermore, RA often goes into remission during pregnancy and flares-up postpartum; its symptoms may be ameliorated and its progression slowed by the use of oral contraceptives (Alexander & LaRosa, 1994; Kiecolt-Glaser & Glaser, 1988). Animal studies have provided support for the role of gonadal hormones in autoimmunity (Ollier & Symmons, 1992).

Genetic and environmental factors are also important contributors to the development of autoimmune disorders. Relatives of patients with autoimmune disorders tend to show a higher than expected incidence of the same disorders, and the prevalence is higher in monozygotic than in dizygotic twins (Merck Research Laboratories, 1992). The prevalence of some autoimmune disorders varies by ethnicity and geographic region. SLE is more common among women of African and Chinese descent (Ollier & Symmons, 1992); it occurs three times more often in African American than in European American women (Carr, 1986). RA is less common among rural Blacks (Ollier & Symmons, 1992) and more common among some Native American groups, such as the Chippewa and Yakima (Weiner, 1991), than among other population groups. MS is five times more frequent in temperate than in tropical climates (Merck Research Laboratories, 1992). Grave's disease is more common in developed countries, and pernicious anemia is more common in northern Europe than in other areas (Ollier & Symmons, 1992). Scleroderma has been found in clusters around airports, which has led to the suggestion that exposure to airplane fuel may be a risk factor (Ollier & Symmons, 1992). Among other suspected toxins under investigation as triggers of autoimmunity are hair dyes (Liang et al., 1991), silicone breast implants (Coleman et al., 1994), and vinyl chloride (Ollier & Symmons, 1992).

Autoimmune disorders tend to have diffuse symptoms, which make them difficult to diagnose. Various autoimmune disorders are often mistaken for one another, and patients may have a long wait before a differential diagnosis can be made. The course of the disorders is unpredictable and idiosyncratic. Some patients experience mild symptoms with little progression, whereas others experience severe symptoms that result in increasing pain and progressive physical deterioration and disability. Patients must expect periods of active disease, which alternate with spontaneous improvement or even remission of symptoms. The unpredictability of autoimmune disorders, the knowledge that the disorders are progressive and incurable, the possibility of deleterious treatment side effects, and the general public's unfamiliarity with most autoimmune disorders can make living with one a frustrating and isolating experience (Chrisler & Parrett, 1995).

CONCERNS OF WOMEN WITH AUTOIMMUNE DISORDERS

Like other people with chronic illnesses, women with autoimmune disorders experience fears about what the future holds (especially with life-threatening and disabling diseases such as SLE and MS), anxiety about undergoing medical treatments or learning the results of medical tests, worry about whether their symptoms will be manageable during upcoming important events, and depression (especially during flare-ups of painful diseases such as RA). Empathic listening, relaxation training, and the teaching of active coping techniques can be very helpful. Cognitive therapy techniques are also useful for clients with chronic illnesses, although therapists should be aware that, especially early on in the person's experience with the disorder, it can be difficult to tell when one's fears and worries are exaggerated. Other concerns are discussed below in the context of life with autoimmune disease.

Adjustment

The diagnosis of a chronic illness is a life-changing event. Gone is the sense of invulnerability so common in youth. People may react to the diagnosis by falling into the familiar *sick role,* which they have often played before when they experienced the flu, chicken pox, or a bad cold. The primary characteristics of the sick role are physical dependency, emotional neediness, and a strong motivation to get well (Lubkin, 1995). However, it is not psychologically healthy (except possibly during flare-ups) to adopt the sick role if one has a chronic illness. Patients with autoimmune disorders are not going to get well, and they would do better to adopt what Gordon (1966) has termed *the impaired role,* in which one strives to maintain normal behavior and responsibilities within the limits of the health condition. Rather than being motivated to recover, patients are motivated to make the most of their abilities. Learning to recognize symptoms, to prevent and manage flare-ups, and to discover one's limits are major tasks of the adjustment period. Other tasks include: learning to carry out one's treatment regimen, adjusting one's work and social schedules, learning to deal with unpredictable situations, adapting to physical disability or deterioration, and normalizing the situation as much as possible (Strauss et al., 1984).

Feminist therapists can help women with autoimmune disorders adjust to the impaired role, which includes incorporating the illness into the self concept without letting it define the self. Therapists can help women realize that they cannot do everything they used to do, nor do they need to do it all. Women can be helped to reorganize their routines; for example, they can learn to do more when they feel well so that they won't feel guilty or fall so far behind when they do less because they feel ill. Some women may need assistance in learning to ask for help when they need it; others may need assistance in learning to do as much as they can for themselves rather than routinely displaying helplessness. Referrals to self-help groups are often appropriate during the adjustment phase.

Physician/Patient Relationships

Physicians' attitudes directly affect the quality of care women receive as well as their ability to make informed decisions about their treatment options (Chrisler & Hemstreet, 1995). The ability of physicians to listen carefully to patients and to see them as experts on their own physical conditions may be particularly important in the case of autoimmune disorders, which are so difficult to diagnose (Chrisler & O'Hea, 2000). This type of consultation and power sharing may be especially unlikely to occur with SLE patients because the physician is most often a White man and the patient most often a Woman of Color (Whitehead, 1992). The pervasive beliefs among physicians that women invent complaints in order to get attention (Fidell, 1980), that women over-report pain (Lack, 1982), and that the vague symptoms that signal the beginning of MS or rheumatic disease are the results of mental, rather than physical, illness can lead physicians to dismiss women's initial complaints, thus delaying proper diagnosis and treatment. In her wide-ranging interviews with women who were living with various chronic illnesses, Marris (1996) found that many of them described their relationships with their physicians, especially in the early stages, as a classic approach-avoidance dilemma. They had to have the cooperation of their physicians if they were ever going to get the help they needed, yet at times the physicians seemed more like enemies than allies.

The likelihood that the physician is male and, by virtue of expertise, in a superior role may subtly encourage women to adopt the traditional feminine role during interactions with health care providers (Chrisler & Hemstreet, 1995). In fact, the role of the patient closely resembles the stereotypic feminine gender role (Williams, 1977). The good patient is passive, cooperative, dependent, uncomplaining, and willing to suffer in silence. Those who complain about their symptoms or treatment or ask a lot of questions are labeled demanding, bad patients, and may be punished by medical staff by being made to wait for treatment or by having their complaints dismissed as hysterical (Chrisler & Hemstreet, 1995). Physicians equate trust in their judgment with being a good patient; therefore, patients who ask a lot of questions or seek alternate opinions are perceived as doubting their physicians' expertise and challenging their judgment (Waitzkin & Waterman, 1974; Wright & Morgan, 1990). Women who are assertive or challenge their physicians are probably more likely than men who behave similarly to be labeled demanding, bad patients. Yet, women with the vague, diffuse symptoms of the early stages of an autoimmune disorder may not get an accurate diagnosis unless they run the risk of annoying their physicians (Chrisler & O'Hea, 2000).

If clients complain about experiencing dismissive treatment from medical personnel, feminist therapists should validate the experience and talk about the sexism, stereotypes, and gender role constraints that underlie the behavior. If the physician's behavior is egregious, encourage the client to find another doctor who will treat her with respect. However, this may be impossible due to managed care regulations or the relative lack of physicians in the area who have expertise and experience with the particular illness. Therapists can assist their clients in finding ways to work with the physician to get their needs met. Clients can be encouraged to write down in advance the questions they want to ask so that they will not become flustered and forget or be silenced before they can ask. Some physicians are annoyed by the sight of a patient with a list of questions, and they may try to end the appointment by walking away before the patient can complete the list. Nurse-psychotherapist Alyce Huston Hemstreet (personal communication, March 2000) teaches her clients to grab the physician's coat pocket as he (or she) walks by and make an assertive statement such as "I'm not finished yet. I need a few more minutes of your time." Faced with the options of risking ripped clothing or sitting down again, most physicians will do the latter. Another good option is for patients to form relationships with nurses or physician's assistants who work in the doctor's practice. These staff members can be important allies; they may be more willing to take the time to explain things to patients, and patients who find their doctors intimidating might be more comfortable calling the nurse or PA to ask a question.

Stress

Stress has repeatedly been shown to compromise immune functioning (Kiecolt-Glaser & Glaser, 1991), and it has been identified as a potential triggering factor in autoimmune disorders (Achterberg-Lawlis, 1982), i.e., stress may exacerbate symptoms or trigger flare-ups. Patients with RA (Affleck, Pfeiffer, Tennen, & Fifeld, 1987) and SLE (Kinash, 1983) have noted that psychological stress triggers their disease flare-ups, and they have reported frequent use of stress management techniques. In one study (Wekking, Vingerhoets, van Dam, Nossent, & Swaak, 1991) the researchers discovered that as the number of reported stressors increased, the physical ability of people with SLE decreased, although the same relationship did not hold for RA patients.

Living with the fatigue, pain, and uncertainties that autoimmune disorders bring adds a layer of stress to those already present in women's lives. Feminist therapists can help their clients to understand their medical conditions as both a cause and effect of stress. Women can be helped to see how the stress of the illness interacts with other already existing stressors, such as daily hassles, financial insecurity, role overload, domestic violence, and struggles with sexism, racism, ethnic prejudice, homophobia, and discrimination based on social class, age, or physical ability. Results of recent research (Klonoff & Landrine, 1995; Landrine, Klonoff, Gibbs, Manning, & Lund, 1995) indicate that Women of Color experience more direct sexism than White women do and that the amount of sexism experienced is related to changes in physical and mental health. There is every reason to assume that being the target of other types of prejudice and discrimination would have similar health effects. Furthermore, physical injuries that result from partner abuse or other violence may produce tissue damage that can trigger autoimmunity (Chrisler & O'Hea, 2000).

Therapists should teach their clients relaxation techniques and other stress management strategies. Women who resist taking time away from family, friends, and community or work responsibilities in order to fit time for relaxation into their schedules can be encouraged to do so by a reminder that they must take care of themselves so that they will be able to take care of others. Life changes (e.g., avoiding interactions that produce tension, working fewer hours, asking for help, dropping less important activities) should also be discussed and evaluated. Clients can be helped to see that many tasks in their daily lives are choices that can be traded off; for example, dropping less important activities can make it possible to conserve the energy necessary to maintain participation in more important activities.

Role Obligations

The symptoms of autoimmune disorders can make it difficult for women to meet the demands of their multiple roles. Interference with role functioning affects patients' relationships with family, friends, and co-workers, as well as their sense of well-being and quality of life (Chrisler & Parrett, 1995). Increasing disability may eventually result in the loss of valued roles, but well-meaning relatives and health care providers may urge women to give up employment or other social roles too soon (Karasz, Bochnak, & Ouellette,

1993), perhaps under the misguided belief that employment is less important to the self-esteem of women than it is to men. The unpredictability of flare-ups and the nature of symptoms (e.g., fatigue, weakness, pain) may make it difficult for women with autoimmune disorders to keep their jobs, especially if they work in pink or blue collar occupations (e.g., clerical, factory, child care jobs), which have the least autonomy and the lowest wages (Shaul, 1994). Educated, skilled workers in white collar occupations who can control the pace and conditions of their work and whose employers are willing to adjust job requirements or work environments are most likely to remain employed after being diagnosed with RA or MS (Gulick, 1992; Yelin, Meenan, Nevitt, & Epstein, 1980). Therapists can help women with autoimmune disorders to consider the impact of their illnesses on their work roles, decide whether and when to inform employers about their conditions, and rehearse asking for changes in duties that would facilitate remaining on the job.

Chronic illness also affects parenting and homemaking roles. Reisine, Goodenow, and Grady (1987) studied women with RA and found that although those who were employed outside the home were less disabled than those who were not, all continued to assume primary responsibility for housework. Allaire (1992) found that little paid household help is used by RA patients, even among those with high incomes. The household tasks most commonly affected by RA flare-ups are cleaning, straightening up, laundry, cooking, and shopping (Reisine et al., 1987). Mothers with RA worry that their symptoms will interfere with parenting, especially with making arrangements, maintaining family ties, and caring for sick children (Reisine et al., 1987), and women report considerable emotional distress when illness affects parenting (Lanza & Revenson, 1993). As it becomes increasingly difficult for women with chronic illness to attend to family and household responsibilities, these are displaced onto family (Allaire, 1992) and friends, which can strain relationships and lead to guilt and anger (Chrisler & Parrett, 1995).

Feminist therapists can help women to understand the gendered nature of the division of household responsibilities and to evaluate the reasonableness of their "need" to do it all. Women who can afford to pay for assistance and services (e.g., child care, housecleaning, grocery delivery) should be encouraged to do so when necessary. Others may be eligible for community services, such as Meals on Wheels, and all can learn to lower their standards (e.g., endure dust longer, serve more frozen foods). Therapists can help women to form a network of relatives, friends, and neighbors in order to avoid depending too much on any one person. Women can also learn to negotiate with partners and children and to provide them with clear explanations about the need for them to do more at certain times. If clients are experiencing resistance from family members at home, some family therapy sessions may be helpful to the client and her partner. Living with someone who has an unpredictable disease and worrying about her pain and disability is stressful, and partners with good social support networks have been found to be less depressed and better able to cope than those who don't (Revenson & Majerovitz, 1991).

Stigma and Isolation

Goffman (1963) defined stigma as undesirable attributes that differ from those we expect in an individual; a discrepancy between expectation and reality can spoil the individual's social identity. Chronic illness may not spoil the identity of an elderly person because chronic illnesses are common, and thus not unexpected, in later life. However, health and vigor are expected of young and middle-aged adults who are assumed to be in the prime of life during the time when autoimmune disorders are most likely to be diagnosed. Therefore, admitting that one has an autoimmune disorder can result in harmful stigmatization (Chrisler & O'Hea, 2000).

The impact of stigma can take various forms (Lubkin, 1995). Healthy individuals may avoid acknowledgment of the existence of the autoimmune disorder either because they do not want to embarrass the individual who is ill or because they want to convey that they do not define the individual in terms of the disease. Individuals who are ill may experience the lack of acknowledgment as silencing or marginalizing. Healthy individuals may also be concerned about making unrealistic demands on their ill co-workers or friends, and thus may leave them out of invitations to social events or opportunities to work on projects. Individuals who are ill may also be left out of groups because healthy people are uncertain about how to behave around them and thus feel uncomfortable in their presence. Repeated experiences of being left out result in social isolation, which contributes to depression. Women with MS (Walsh & Walsh, 1989) and RA (Goodenow, Reisine, & Grady, 1990) have been found to make and receive fewer visits from friends, and they experience feelings of isolation, in part because they know few others in their situation.

Stigma may also result from disorders that have invisible symptoms. Healthy people may assume that people with autoimmune disorders are fine when they are not because they look normal. Tiredness, weakness, and pain are common to many of the autoimmune disorders, and these can be difficult to describe to others. We all get tired; in fact, many women are fatigued much of the time due to their many roles (Marris, 1996). These symptoms may be categorized by healthy people as illegitimate (Thornton & Lea, 1992), and people with invisible symptoms may be labeled as complainers.

Symptom flare-ups and decreasing mobility can increase women's sense of isolation as they are forced to spend more time at home. Therapists should be alert for signs of depression, especially in times of role transition such as loss of employment. Friendships at work are often a major part of an individual's social life, and it may prove difficult to maintain these once the work ties are broken (Chrisler & O'Hea, 2000). Clients may benefit from referrals to support groups for people with their particular diagnosis with whom they can discuss these issues. They can also be helped to understand the process of stigmatization, to form more accurate attributions for the behavior of healthy people, to educate others about their disorders, and to learn to tell people how they want to be treated (e.g., "Please continue to invite me to events. Let me decide whether or not I can attend."). Women whose symptoms affect their mobility should be encouraged to get "handicapped" tags for their cars and to try mobility assistance devices (e.g., motorized scooters) so that they need not remain isolated at home.

Body Image and Sexuality

Although psychological research on body image concerns has been largely confined to studies of adolescents and disordered eaters, body image issues can arise at any age and are likely to be associated with chronic, debilitating disorders (Chrisler & Ghiz, 1993). Body image concerns can be expected to emerge in women with autoimmune disorders as increasing fatigue, weakness, pain, and joint deformity alter appearance and mobility (Chrisler & Parrett, 1995). Medication side effects and changes in activity level due to symptom severity may lead to weight gain, which can also trigger body image concerns. Feminist therapists should be alert to their clients' concerns about bodily changes and work with them in much the same way that they would with healthy clients. Women who are mourning their inability to continue athletic pursuits may be helped by encouragement to try new activities that don't stress their joints or require the same degree of flexibility; for example, tennis players or joggers might try swimming, water aerobics, or yoga.

Sexuality concerns have not been well studied in women with autoimmune disorders, and most researchers have tended to emphasize a woman's ability to be an effective sexual partner for a man rather than her ability to meet her own needs (Chrisler & Parrett, 1995). Sexual dysfunctions have been found to occur frequently in MS patients. Increased dysfunction is generally correlated with increased disability, and MS patients report being troubled by fatigue, decreased sensation and libido, insufficient orgasm, and low arousability (Stenager, Stenager, Jensen, & Boldson, 1990). Women with RA and SLE most commonly mention pain or weakness, fatigue, and problems with their partners as interfering with sexual activity (Ferguson & Figley, 1979). As many physicians are uncomfortable talking about sexual activity with their patients, feminist therapists can be helpful by asking women with autoimmune disorders if they have any concerns about sexuality. If the answer is yes, standard sex therapy techniques may be useful, as might an exploration of what it means to be sexual and encouragement to try new, possibly more physically comfortable, positions and activities.

Because of the relatively young ages at which some autoimmune disorders are diagnosed, feminist therapists may be called upon to support women as they make reproductive decisions. Miscarriage rates are high among lupus patients (Newell & Coeshott, 1998), and flare-ups are common during pregnancy and postpartum (Achterberg-Lawlis, 1988; Kiecolt-Glaser & Glaser, 1988). Women with lupus, MS, and RA often worry that increasing disability may make it difficult for them to manage child care activities. Clients should be encouraged to gather information from medical professionals and from disease foundations and to ask women in support groups about their experiences. Feminist therapists can help their clients to sort through the ramifications of their decisions, including dealing with feelings of loss should they decide that having children is too risky.

CONCLUSION

Women with autoimmune disorders can benefit from psychotherapy as they adjust to their diagnosis and learn to cope with their symptoms. Support for grief reactions and identity changes can be offered from any philosophical approach. Feminist therapists can also help women with chronic illness through crisis management; techniques for anxiety, stress, anger, and pain management; assertiveness training; and coping with uncertainty and fear of death or disability (Goodheart & Lansing, 1997). Encouragement to keep a journal or the use of other literary or art therapy techniques can also be helpful to women with chronic illness in coming to terms with their situations.

Feminist therapists who work with women with autoimmune disorders do not need to be medical experts on the various disorders, but they should do some general reading about women's health (e.g., Blechman & Brownell, 1998; Dan, 1994; Stanton & Gallant, 1995) and behavioral medicine (e.g., Camic & Knight, 1998; Goodheart & Lansing, 1997). First hand accounts, such as disability activist Nancy Mairs' (1996) accounts of living with MS and excerpts of Veronica Marris' (1996) interviews with women with chronic illness, are very helpful in understanding the issues that women with chronic illnesses must confront, and these can also be suggested to clients as bibliotherapy. The disease foundations (e.g., Lupus Foundation of America, Multiple Sclerosis Association of America, United Scleroderma Foundation) are excellent sources of information that is written for lay readers, and they all have web sites on the internet for quick access. It's useful to have a copy of the Merck Manual (Merck Research Laboratories, 1992) available to read brief explanations of medical conditions. Any further information that may be necessary can be gained by asking the clients about their conditions or by requesting their permission to speak to their physicians.

Therapists should also assemble a list of referral sources, such as local self-help groups and mailing addresses, phone numbers, and internet addresses of the major disease foundations. Women with mobility problems who have access to the internet might like to make use of chat rooms that function as support groups, and they should be encouraged to try them. Finally, feminist therapists with an interest in chronic illness and some experience working with women with autoimmune disorders could provide a service to the community by offering to provide meeting space, group facilitation, and psychoeducational training for women who could benefit from group work and social support.

REFERENCES

Achterberg-Lawlis, J. (1988). Musculoskeletal disorders. In E. A. Blechman & K. D. Brownell (Eds.), *Handbook of behavioral medicine for women* (pp. 222-235). New York: Pergamon.

Affleck, G., Pfeiffer, C., Tennen, H., & Fifield, J. (1987). Attributional processes in rheumatoid arthritis patients. *Arthritis and Rheumatism, 30,* 927-931.

Alexander, L. L., & LaRosa, J. H. (1994). *New dimensions in women's health.* Boston: Jones & Bartlett.

Allaire, S. H. (1992). Employment and household work disability in women with rheumatoid arthritis. *Journal of Applied Rehabilitation Counseling, 23,* 44-51.

Blechman, E. A., & Brownell, K. D. (Eds.). (1998). *Behavioral medicine & women: A comprehensive handbook.* New York: Guilford.

Camic, P., & Knight, S. (Eds.). (1998). *Clinical handbook of health psychology.* Seattle: Hogrefe & Huber.

Carlson, K., Eisenstat, S., & Ziporyn, T. (1996). *The Harvard guide to women's health.* Cambridge, MA: Harvard University Press.

Carr, R. (1986). *Lupus erythematosus: A handbook for physicians, patients, and their families.* Rockville, MD: Lupus Foundation of America.

Chrisler, J. C., & Ghiz, L. (1993). Body image issues of older women. *Women & Therapy, 14*(1/2), 67-75.

Chrisler, J. C., & Hemstreet, A. H. (1995). The diversity of women's health needs. In J. C. Chrisler & A. H. Hemstreet (Eds.), *Variations on a theme: Diversity and the psychology of women* (pp. 1-28). Albany, NY: State University of New York Press.

Chrisler, J. C., & O'Hea, E. L. (2000). Gender, culture, and autoimmune disorders. In R. M. Eisler & M. Hersen (Eds.), *Handbook of gender, culture, and health* (pp. 321-342). Mahwah, NJ: Erlbaum.

Chrisler, J. C., & Parrett, K. L. (1995). Women and autoimmune disorders. In A. L. Stanton & S. J. Gallant (Eds.), *The psychology of women's health: Progress and challenges in research and application* (pp. 171-195). Washington, DC: APA Books.

Coleman, E. A., Lemon, S. J., Rudick, J., Depuy, R. S., Feuer, E. J., & Edwards, B. K. (1994). Rheumatic disease among 1167 women reporting local implant and systemic problems after breast implant surgery. *Journal of Women's Health, 3,* 165-177.

Crowley, L. V. (1997). *Introduction to human disease* (4th ed.). Sudbury, MA: Jones & Bartlett.

Dan, A. (Ed.). (1994). *Reframing women's health: Multidisciplinary research and practice.* Newbury Park, CA: Sage.

Falvo, D. R. (1991). *Medical and psychosocial aspects of chronic illness and disability.* Gaithersburg, MD: Aspen.

Ferguson, K., & Figley, B. (1979). Sexuality and rheumatic disease: A prospective study. *Sexuality & Disability, 2,* 130-138.

Fidell, L. S. (1980). Sex role stereotypes and the American physician. *Psychology of Women Quarterly, 4,* 313-330.

Goffman, E. (1963). *Stigma: Notes on management of spoiled identity.* Englewood Cliffs, NJ: Prentice Hall.

Goodenow, C., Reisine, S. T., & Grady, K. E. (1990). Quality of social support and associated social and psychological functioning in women with rheumatoid arthritis. *Health Psychology, 9,* 266-284.

Goodheart, C. D., & Lansing, M. H. (1997). *Treating people with chronic illness: A psychological guide.* Washington, DC: APA Books.

Gordon, G. (1966). *Role theory and illness: A sociological perspective.* New Haven, CT: College and University Press.

Gulick, E. E. (1992). Model for predicting work performance among persons with multiple sclerosis. *Nursing Research, 41,* 266-272.

Karasz, A. K., Bochnak, E., & Ouellette, S. C. (1993, August). *Role strain and psychological well-being in lupus patients.* Paper presented at the meeting of the American Psychological Association, Toronto, Canada.

Kiecolt-Glaser, J. K., & Glaser, R. (1988). Immunological competence. In E. A. Blechman & K. D. Brownell (Eds.), *Handbook of behavioral medicine for women* (pp. 195-205). New York: Pergamon.

Kiecolt-Glaser, J. K., & Glaser, R. (1991). Stress and immune function in humans. In R. Ader, D. Felton, & N. Cohen (Eds.), *Psychoneuroimmunology* (pp. 849-867). New York: Academic Press.

Kinash, R. G. (1983, June). Systemic lupus erythematosus: The psychological dimension. *Canada's Mental Health, 31,* 19-22.

Klonoff, E. A., & Landrine, H. (1995). The Schedule of Sexist Events: A measure of life-time and recent sexist discrimination in women's lives. *Psychology of Women Quarterly, 19,* 439-472.

Knight, S. J., & Camic, P. M. (1998). Health psychology and medicine: The art and science of healing. In Camic, P. & Knight, S. (Eds.), *Clinical handbook of health psychology* (pp. 3-15). Seattle: Hogrefe & Huber.

Lack, D. Z. (1982). Women and pain: Another feminist issue. *Women & Therapy, 1*(1), 55-64.

Landrine, H., Klonoff, E. A., Gibbs, J., Manning, V., & Lund, M. (1995). Physical and psychiatric correlates of gender discrimination: An application of the Schedule of Sexist Events. *Psychology of Women Quarterly, 19,* 473-492.

Lanza, A. F., & Revenson, T. A. (1993, August). *Rheumatic diseases, social roles, and the social support matching hypothesis.* Paper presented at the meeting of the American Psychological Association, Toronto, Canada.

Liang, M., Partridge, A., Daltroy, L., Straaton, K., Galper, S., & Holman, H. (1991). Strategies for reducing excess morbidity and mortality in Blacks with systemic lupus erythematosus. *Arthritis and Rheumatism, 34,* 1187-1196.

Lubkin, I. M. (1995). *Chronic illness: Impact and interventions* (3rd ed.). Sudbury, MA: Jones & Bartlett.

Mairs, N. (1996). *Waist high in the world: A life among the nondisabled.* Boston: Beacon.

Marris, V. (1996). *Lives worth living: Women's experience of chronic illness.* London: HarperCollins.

Merck Research Laboratories. (1992). *The Merck manual of diagnosis and therapy* (16th ed.). Rahway, NJ: Merck & Co.

Newell, M. K., & Coeshott, C. (1998). Lupus. In E. A. Blechman & K. D. Brownell (Eds.), *Behavioral medicine & women: A comprehensive handbook* (pp. 682-687). New York: Guilford.

Ollier, W., & Symmons, D. P. M. (1992). *Autoimmunity.* Oxford: BIOS Scientific.

Reisine, S. T., Goodenow, C., & Grady, K. E. (1987). The impact of rheumatoid arthritis on the homemaker. *Social Science and Medicine, 25,* 89-95.

Revenson, T. A., & Majerovitz, S. D. (1991). The effects of chronic illness on the spouse: Social resources as stress buffers. *Arthritis Care and Research, 4,* 63-72.

Shaul, M. P. (1994). Rheumatoid arthritis and older women: Economics tell only part of the story. *Health Care for Women International, 15,* 377-383.

Stanton, A. L., & Gallant, S. J. (Eds.). (1995). *The psychology of women's health: Progress and challenges in research and application.* Washington, DC: APA Books.

Stenager, E., Stenager, E. N., Jensen, K., & Boldsen, J. (1990). Multiple sclerosis: Sexual dysfunctions. *Journal of Sex Education and Therapy, 16,* 262-269.

Strauss, A. L., Corbin, J., Fagerhaugh, S., Glaser, B., Maines, D., Suczek, B., & Wiener, C. (1984). *Chronic illness and the quality of life.* St. Louis: Mosby.

Taylor, S. E. (1999). *Health psychology* (4th ed.). New York: McGraw-Hill.

Thornton, H. B., & Lea, S. J. (1992). An investigation into needs of people living with multiple sclerosis and their families. *Disability, Handicap, & Society, 7,* 321-338.

Waitzkin, H. B., & Waterman, B. (1974). *The exploitation of illness in capitalist society.* Indianapolis: Bobbs-Merrill.

Walsh, A., & Walsh, P. A. (1989). Love, self-esteem, and multiple sclerosis. *Social Science and Medicine, 29,* 793-798.

Weiner, H. (1991). Social and psychobiological factors in autoimmune disease. In R. Ader, D. Felton, & N. Cohen (Eds.), *Psychoneuroimmunology* (pp. 955-1011). New York: Academic Press.

Wekking, E. M., Vingerhoets, A. J., van Dam, A. P., Nossent, J. C., & Swaak, A. J.

(1991). Daily stressors and systemic lupus erythematosus: A longitudinal analysis–first findings. *Psychotherapy and Psychosomatics, 55,* 108-113.

Whitehead, K. (1992). Systemic lupus erythematosus: Another woman's problem? *Feminism & Psychology, 2,* 189-195.

William, J. H. (1977). *Psychology of women: Behavior in a biosocial context.* New York: Norton.

Wright, A. L., & Morgan, W. J. (1990). On the creation of "problem" patients. *Social Science and Medicine, 30,* 951-959.

Yellin, E., Meenan, R., Nevitt, M., & Epstein, W. (1980). Work disability in rheumatoid arthritis: Effects of disease, social, and work factors. *Annals of Internal Medicine, 93,* 551-556.

Chronic Fatigue Syndrome:
A First-Person Story

Paula J. Caplan

SUMMARY. Real physical illnesses are often misinterpreted and misdiagnosed as psychological or at least as psychogenic problems, especially in women and especially when the illness is not well understood.
This is a first-person story about the author's history of what ultimately
was diagnosed as Chronic Fatigue Syndrome. The frustrating political,
social, medical, and economic contexts of living with this syndrome are
described on the basis of the author's experience, and suggestions are
offered for therapists working with people who suffer from or may
suffer from this and similar medical problems. *[Article copies available
for a fee from The Haworth Document Delivery Service: 1-800-342-9678.
E-mail address: <getinfo@haworthpressinc.com> Website: <http://www.Haworth
Press.com> © 2001 by The Haworth Press, Inc. All rights reserved.]*

KEYWORDS. Chronic Fatigue Syndrome, chronic fatigue immune
deficiency syndrome, fibromyalgia, multiple chemical sensitivities

CLUELESS IN TORONTO

Beware: Being a therapist can be dangerous to your physical and mental
health. You may misinterpret as psychogenic problems that in fact are physi-

Paula J. Caplan, PhD, is an affiliated scholar at Brown University's Pembroke
Center.

Address correspondence to: Paula J. Caplan, PhD, Pembroke Center, Brown
University, Box 1958, Providence, RI 02912.

[Haworth co-indexing entry note]: "Chronic Fatigue Syndrome: A First-Person Story." Caplan, Paula
J. Co-published simultaneously in *Women & Therapy* (The Haworth Press, Inc.) Vol. 23, No. 1, 2001, pp. 23-43;
and: *Minding the Body: Psychotherapy in Cases of Chronic and Life-Threatening Illness* (ed: Ellyn
Kaschak) The Haworth Press, Inc., 2001, pp. 23-43. Single or multiple copies of this article are available for
a fee from The Haworth Document Delivery Service [1-800-342-9678, 9:00 a.m. - 5:00 p.m. (EST). E-mail
address: getinfo@haworthpressinc.com].

cal. I am a clinical and research psychologist, and while teaching graduate students for years I had noticed two things about myself. On days when I taught, I avoided planning to do anything that wasn't absolutely necessary the rest of the day and evening because I knew I would have a splitting headache, the pain from which would probably wake me, nauseated, in the middle of the night. Bringing my psychological training to bear, I thought, "Isn't it funny? I *thought* I loved teaching, but obviously, at least unconsciously, I don't, because I get a stress headache every time I teach." Mentioning these headaches to my physician brought no suggestions beyond my own interpretation. Similarly, I observed that, increasingly, at break time during the three-hour seminars, I would seek out a student and ask (feeling foolish), "Am I making any sense today?" The answer was invariably "Yes," but again using my psychological approach, I concluded, "I *thought* I had some confidence in my teaching ability, but clearly I don't, because my insecurity compels me to ask repeatedly for reassurance." This went on for years.

I had long been alarmed by the damage done when normal behavior, especially in women, is pathologized and when normal, healthy behavior and human fear, depression, confusion, and anguish are unjustifiably attributed to biological/chemical differences and treated in knee-jerk fashion with psychotropic drugs, electroshock, and surgery (e.g., Caplan, 2000, 1995, 1994, 1992, 1991; Caplan & Gans, 1991; Caplan, McCurdy-Myers, & Gans, 1992; Pantony & Caplan, 1991). I had put considerable time and energy into research, writing, public education, and organizing of social action in regard to these concerns. Until now, I have not written about the misinterpretation of real physical problems, especially in women, as psychological . . . and psychopathological. Without my knowing it, for many years the latter was exactly what was happening to me. Perhaps most disturbingly, I, too, misinterpreted physiologically-based problems as psychological because of my lack of knowledge first about the very existence and later about the nature of what is now variously called "Chronic Fatigue Syndrome," "Chronic Fatigue Immune Dysfunction Syndrome," "Multiple Chemical Sensitivity," "Fibromyalgia," and various other things outside of North America.

It took me many years to realize that my headaches and confusion were connected to a wide variety of other problems for which I had sought treatment over the years, including feelings of sleepiness and exhaustion that never left me, a large and increasing number of allergies or sensitivities to foods (even to apples and rice, foods to which I was told no one is allergic) and chemicals. In traffic jams, for instance, I would feel desperately ill from breathing diesel fumes, whereas if I closed the air vent in my car the symptoms would lessen. Traffic jams had not previously made me feel *that* ill. I also experienced severe fluid retention, steadily increasing weight–especially around my middle, which one hears indicates heart-attack risk–and exhaustion after even slight physical exertion.

As a feminist, I felt that worrying about weight for cosmetic reasons was shameful, but I was repeatedly told that my back, hip, and foot pains were caused or exacerbated by my weight, and that did worry me. I was swept along by a culture whose members variously told me I was just working too hard, not *trying* to relax, being hypochondriacal, eating the wrong things (I systematically stopped eating *everything* that seemed to make me feel worse), not exercising enough (they looked askance when I said truthfully that on any day when I spent 40 minutes at low to moderate speed on the treadmill, I would have to go to bed and stay there as soon as I got home), needed cranial-sacral adjustments, needed a really *good* acupuncturist (I paid a lot of money to the best chiropractors, massage therapists, and acupuncturists in Toronto for years, getting little or no relief), needed to go on the anti-yeast diet (I did, many times, to little or no effect), and on and on and on.

When I took my children on a trip that included climbing a bit of a slope, everyone else in the group, from kids to people 40 years older than I, walked straight to the top, getting there long before me. When I finally caught up with them, I felt as though my chest were going to explode. I was frustrated and embarrassed, assuming that proved I was in terrible shape due to lack of self-discipline. I didn't seem to be wheezing, so the possibility of asthma never entered my mind. Also, the first time I had had trouble breathing deeply was around the time my children's father and I were divorcing, so my friends and I assumed that the breathing problem was psychogenic. Checking it out with my physician, I had a chest X-ray that was negative. The doctor said my breathing problem was psychological and, because I was having trouble sleeping, after great resistance from me, urged me to take what was being marketed as a sleeping pill, Halcyon. "Don't worry," he assured me, "it's not like Valium. It has no side effects." Within a day, the Halcyon caused me to be overcome with weeping. I threw the bottle away.

That same physician told me, when I sought treatment for a bad cold, "You probably wouldn't have gotten this cold if you weren't so fat!" Every time I saw this doctor, whom I was reluctant to leave because he seemed to prescribe fewer drugs than most general practitioners, he handed me a diet sheet and told me to lose weight. I conscientiously inspected each new diet and then informed him truthfully, "If I ate this much food, I would weigh more than I weigh now." I had tried eating more, eating less, eating differently in a variety of ways. On one such occasion he looked at me skeptically and said, "You can't eat what you claim to eat. You wouldn't look like this if you did. You must eat peanut butter in bed." I finally got another GP.

Despite its totally draining effect on me, I also assiduously tried exercise, hoping it would increase my stamina, decrease my exhaustion, and maybe alleviate other problems. Religiously, I spent 40 minutes a day on the tread-mill six days a week and alternated upper-body with lower-body weight-bearing exercises. After 18 months of this regime, I had increased my stamina and strength not at all, and my body fat, weight, and fluid retention were unchanged. As Vivienne Anderson (2000) has pointed out, chronically ill people struggle with the myth that people can control their bodies.

THE LIGHT BEGINS TO DAWN

That's a brief summary of my symptoms over nearly two decades. But let us return to the early 1990s, when I connected only the symptoms of head-ache and confusion, which I later learned are called "brain fog" and feel like being on high doses of antihistamines, with my teaching. One summer, I had the idea to meet with my thesis and dissertation supervisees at my home rather than in the building where I taught and had my office, the Ontario Institute for Studies in Education (OISE), the graduate faculty of education of the University of Toronto. That summer, I entered the building only a couple of times a week, just long enough to take the elevator to the ninth floor, walk to my mailbox, speak briefly to my secretary, take the mail, and leave. That summer, I had no headaches; interestingly, I never noticed. When September came, the first day back in the building I developed a splitting headache, and then it registered: maybe something in the building is causing the problem.

A few days later, while twelve students in one of my seminars watched a short film, I took out a small kit for measuring carbon monoxide levels and checked the air in the seminar room. When the film ended, I explained what I had been doing and why. I had not found the carbon monoxide level to be elevated, but ten of the twelve students said that something must be wrong, because they experienced moderate to severe respiratory problems and/or severe headaches when and only when in that building. One graduate student in nursing said, "I can spend eight hours in the nursing building with no problem, but for several hours after I leave the OISE building, I have breathing problems and congestion." Another confessed that she had been morti-fied about leaving class every day at the 90-minute break, but she had no choice because of the pain from her migraine headaches. I had assumed that she was bored by my teaching. I learned that "brain fog" is a frequent consequence of toxic air and was what had led me to ask students if my lectures were making sense.

After that first September headache, more things began to click for me. I started to recall that people who worked in the OISE building had always made jokes about its bad air. OISE's 12-story building is sealed; you cannot open a window, and only a small proportion of the air that is brought in is fresh. Like many buildings constructed in recent decades, it was built that way to save on energy, not a bad idea in and of itself if it did no harm. I had actually assumed that a sealed building would be good for my hay fever because it would reduce the pollen in my office. At that time, during the early 1990s in Toronto, no one I knew thought seriously that "bad air," whatever that meant in an academic building (not a factory, after all!) in a supposedly civilized country could cause health problems. A senior woman faculty member who had helped pioneer women's studies there was known to have something that was beginning to be called "Chronic Fatigue" and was only working part-time. But not until months after that September headache did I even begin to wonder whether my own chronic exhaustion might be due to the building's air. It was easy enough to attribute those feelings to being a single mother with a fulltime paid job who was also writing books and articles, giving invited lectures, and doing some public education and other social action work, as well as trying to spend some time with family and friends.

TAKING ACTION

I organized various kinds of protest. I held class on the front steps of the building and called the media to dramatize the fact that it was not healthy to be in the building and that I did not feel comfortable insisting that my students spend hours inside. I wrote letters to and met with members of the Ontario provincial parliament. I wrote to the president of the University of Toronto. Some students and I led a march through the building, chanting concerns about the air; and the students circulated a petition. They stood outside the OISE cafeteria and asked everyone who walked by to sign the petition if and only if they had health problems that they experienced only in the OISE building. People who signed were asked to describe their symptoms. Hundreds of people signed, creating lists of symptoms, and only a handful said they had no reason to sign because they had no symptoms. Some of the latter developed symptoms in later years. I cannot prove this, but it appears to me that nearly everyone who spends long periods of time in the OISE building develops symptoms eventually. It seems that people have varying susceptibilities to toxic air so that some people become symptomatic quite rapidly but others not for years. Everyone is different, some more sensitive than others to the effects of chemical and other (e.g., dust, mold) exposures. A graduate student who ran marathons told me she was pretty comfortable in the OISE building but, unlike in other buildings, at OISE she could not walk up the stairs, because she quickly became winded. Another student had a splitting headache each time she was at OISE, but for her two years there she attributed the headaches to the emotional stress of working on her Master's degree. As soon as her coursework was completed, she took a fulltime job that required far more than forty hours a week and was highly stressful, and she was writing her thesis at the same time. Her headaches returned only when she had to go back to OISE to use the library to work on her thesis.

Employees, mostly women, whose work kept them tied to the building the greatest number of hours per day (usually the lowest-paid workers) would take me aside, saying, "I heard you are trying to get the air in the building cleaned up. Good for you." I would reply, "Oh, do you have any health problems in the building?" They would describe what they experienced, and I would say, "That is so important. Would you please write a letter to the administration about that, with a copy to me?" And then I would hear their stories. They had already reported their complaints, and in many cases the administration's responses had been in one or both of these categories: "This is due to job stress" or "Are you on the rag?" Having had their real health problems thus dismissed or mocked, and often desperately needing those poorly-paid jobs, they had retreated to silence and were afraid to make a fuss.

Despite the hard work of the handful of graduate students who helped in the campaign to bring clean air to OISE, nothing changed. I learned a lot. The building was regularly sprayed with pesticides, but workers were not alerted in advance that spraying was scheduled. As an employee, I had never been informed that pesticides were used at all. The duct system that carries air through the building had never been cleaned in the 25 or more years since the building had been constructed. One faculty member wrote to inquire about this and was told by the administration that that type of duct system could not be cleaned. The faculty member then sent a memo listing the name and phone number of a company that had confirmed that it could indeed clean the OISE system, but by the time I left OISE's employ some years later the ducts had not been cleaned. One of my students knew an expert on building air quality and asked him to check the OISE air. He told me that he had placed a tissue over a vent that brings air into an OISE office, and in twenty minutes black material had accumulated on the tissue. He said that this was a carbon compound and was carcinogenic, and he explained that we were regularly inhaling that air into our lungs.

The same expert also said that any building houses dust, molds, and a variety of chemicals, such as formaldehyde, that is emitted as furniture deteriorates over the years and benzene that is produced as paint ages. A variety of things grow when carpets are shampooed but not thoroughly dried, and all sorts of chemicals are used in regular office work, not to mention emissions from computer terminals. Adequate air ventilation and circulation help keep the molecules of each of these substances from combining with molecules of other substances. When giant molecules made up of these various toxins form and remain in the air, our bodies find it difficult or impossible to break them down. That is why, even when officials report that levels of dust, mold, and chemicals are not particularly high in a given air sample, they may well be high enough to damage people's health. Furthermore, the air quality expert said, significant permanent damage can be done to a person's health if that person is simultaneously exposed to a number of different chemicals, even at relatively low levels. A further complication is that levels of problematic substances may vary from one part of a building to another, so that a test result showing a normal level in one office or on one floor may not be applicable to all others in the same building.

REASONS FOR DISBELIEF

These principles are still not widely known in the population at large, and they were even less familiar during the early 1990s when I was learning about them. This lack of information was, I believe, a primary reason for the powerful resistance of the vast majority of my colleagues to recognizing the problem and their failure to participate in the campaign to improve OISE's air. One professor, a bright and caring teacher, was known for falling asleep during his own lectures. I learned that, because he developed severe allergic symptoms every time he was at OISE, he loaded up on antihistamines whenever he had to teach. He did not participate in the campaign. Like most people, he was accustomed to dealing with standard kinds of allergies and therefore was probably comfortable in treating his symptoms as routine allergic reactions. Indeed, who wants to believe that their workplace is dangerous to their health? Few people have the option to leave their jobs, especially the employees who were most likely to spend long hours in the building, most of whom had the lowest-status and lowest-paid jobs in non-union categories and many of whom were recent immigrants or single mothers.

To this day, as far as I can determine, the air at OISE has not been improved. Each time I meet someone who still works there, I hear about more people who have now been definitively diagnosed as having Chronic Fatigue or who are reporting, as one person told me, being "exhausted all the time." One woman had worked at OISE long before I began teaching there and had seemed to have a particularly strong constitution and excellent health. She told me recently that she attributes her current exhaustion to "job stress." My reply was, "Are you kidding? You have worked under enormous pressure for thirty years. And now you are getting to do a lot more work that you enjoy. Don't you think it is just possible that the problem is physical, caused by the cumulative effect of the poor-quality air?" She did not want to consider that possibility. I recently read a published paper in which a respected scholar reports that she began experiencing extreme fatigue when she first went to work in Toronto. Although she does not mention this, I know that that work was in the OISE building.

Attributing physical problems to job stress or allergies allows one to maintain the illusion of control, the belief that one is not really in danger and is able to protect one's health if one can just learn to relax or avoid milk products or get through ragweed season. Allergies and stress are real and certainly can be dangerous, but they are not the only causes of persistent fatigue or other physical problems.

MORE ATTEMPTS TO IMPEL CHANGE

When I realized that something in the building was consistently doing bad things to my body, that I was not simply afflicted by stress headaches and insecurity, *and* when I realized that the harm went far beyond me, that many people were being affected and it was impossible to know how many were being harmed and to what extent, I decided to do whatever I could to keep both other people and myself out of the building as much as possible. The semester when I realized what was happening, I started holding my seminar course meetings at my home. Many students were glad to avoid the building for those three-hour periods, but some found it extremely inconvenient because they had other courses or work back at OISE just before or just after my course hours or because their children were in daycare near OISE. So the following semester I did my OISE teaching in a room at New College, a University of Toronto college with which I had an affiliation through my work in the undergraduate Women's Studies program there. I simply asked to reserve a New College room regularly during that semester. Its proximity to OISE was a plus, but someone pointed out that the arrangement could lead to major problems of legal liability. If an OISE student were injured at New College, would New College unwittingly be liable? Would I personally be liable for having made this unorthodox arrangement, an arrangement that had not gone through anyone at OISE or through the Principal of New College?

Assuming it would be a simple matter to ask the Director of OISE to send a letter to the New College principal, officially requesting that I be allowed to use the New College space–or, failing that, for the OISE Director to use some of his longstanding contacts in other parts of the University, where he had been a senior administrator just before taking over the OISE directorship, I asked him to do so. He did not. I will not speculate on the reasons that he failed to do so, but within a couple of years the two of us who constituted the core faculty in the Feminist Community Psychology program (both tenured, Full Professors), the only OISE program that had an explicit, feminist, social action component, were gone from OISE.

I had arranged to take a sabbatical. My plan was to remain in Toronto because my daughter was still in high school. Just before I began my sabbatical, I wrote to OISE's Assistant Director for Academic Affairs, enclosing a physician's letter (I was subsequently to send similar letters from other physicians: a general practitioner, an allergy specialist, and a specialist on occupational health) that indicated that something in the building appeared to be harmful to my health. My cover letter included the request that, by the time my sabbatical ended, the OISE administration would have arranged for me to teach and have office space in any University of Toronto building that was not sealed. Repeated letters of inquiry about the status of this request were ignored. In the meantime, I was doing my sabbatical writing and carrying on attempts to ensure that the air in the building would be improved for everyone's sakes.

During the couple of years of the ongoing protest about the OISE air, some strange things happened. Although the OISE administration had sent out a newsletter in which they acknowledged that they were aware that hundreds of people became ill because of the building every day, in interviews with the media they denied that there was any problem. The OISE Occupational Health and Safety Committee took no action to improve the air. It took me many telephone calls to the appropriate government agency of the province of Ontario to get anyone to come out and check the air in the building. After they did, they called a meeting with members of the administration, and I was invited to that meeting, which we held on an outside deck at OISE because of the problems with the air inside the building. The government official explained that the OISE air met provincial air quality standards. However, he went on quite spontaneously to explain that Ontario really had no specific standards for air quality within an *office building,* so they had used the standards for factories. Yes, you read that correctly. He said further that Ontario's standards for air quality were notoriously lax. I was dumbfounded. How could he make that series of statements and then fail utterly to insist that the air be cleaned up? How could OISE fail to conduct an epidemiological study to see how many of its employees and students were being harmed and in what ways? I do not know the answers to these questions, but I find them deeply disturbing. The failure of the OISE and University administrations, members of the Ontario Provincial Parliament, and employees of government agencies to take action is unconscionable.

I had noticed that, despite my absence from the building, I continued to feel overwhelmingly tired and sleepy almost all the time nearly every day. I had begun to wonder whether the increasing numbers of allergies and sensitivities to foods, cigarette smoke, and chemicals which I had been noticing in myself might somehow be related to what I was then calling "Sick Building Syndrome" (Blank, 1998). The headaches and brain fog only returned on the exceedingly rare occasions when I had to spend more than ten minutes in another sealed building. For instance, when I had to give guest or keynote lectures in buildings and, still not realizing that many sealed buildings were "sick," I neglected to check ahead of time to make sure I could speak in a safe, open building, I felt ill. The only times I entered the OISE building during my sabbatical were the occasional visits that lasted just long enough for me to pick up mail or leave papers for my secretary or students. Although by then I suspected that wearing a paper mask over my nose and mouth would not keep out the chemicals that did me the most harm, I wore a mask as a feeble attempt to minimize further risk. Once, in the OISE elevator, a top OISE administrator mocked me in front of a large number of people for wearing the mask. Another time, my secretary overheard a senior OISE person saying, again in a crowded elevator, "Why doesn't Paula Caplan just go work someplace else?" I had headed the Centre for Women's Studies, the School Psychology Program, and the Feminist Community Psychology Program at OISE. It's hard at such times to feel solidly justified in what one is doing and not to feel hurt and ostracized. I tell these incidents here because I have learned how isolated each of a huge number of women and men has felt under similar circumstances.

THE LABELS

For some time, I called my condition "Sick Building Syndrome," a term that referred to its presumed cause. Over many years, I learned that these symptoms are often clustered with the sleep disturbances, muscle pains, allergies/sensitivities, chest pain and constricted breathing, and exhaustion after even mild exercise that I had experienced. These various symptoms also tend to characterize what has been called "Gulf War Syndrome," perhaps because sick buildings and the Gulf War have in common simultaneous exposures to multiple chemicals (Duehring, 1997). The allergies and sensitivities are sometimes called Multiple Chemical Sensitivity or MCS (see the excellent, comprehensive work by Pamela Reed Gibson, including Gibson, 2000; Gibson, Cheavens, & Warren, 1996, 1998), and people diagnosed with MCS often describe their reactions to chemicals as including the kinds of symptoms I have had, which are listed above. The diagnosis of "Fibromyalgia" (Quinn, 1997) refers to the presence of large numbers of muscle aches and sensitive pressure-points, which also are often found in people who have sleep disturbances. In my own case, because I fell asleep easily and slept eight hours a night, it never occurred to me that I had a sleep disorder. Only recently did I realize that my constant exhaustion strongly indicated poor *quality* sleep. Obviously, the original term "Chronic Fatigue Syndrome" refers to the fatigue and energy problems, and people with those problems often experience many or all of the symptoms I have had. The newer term, "Chronic Fatigue Immune Dysfunction Syndrome or CFIDS," refers to presumed malfunctioning of the immune system, for reasons perhaps including but not limited to chemical exposures, which may underlie the symptom picture. Many people with one or more or all of these symptom types have received or will receive one or more or all of the above labels, and many diagnosed with, for instance, MCS, will also report extreme fatigue and/or muscle aches. But a lot of those people, including me, do not match the Chronic Fatigue symptom list selected with rather poor scientific rigor by the Centers for Disease Control (the CDC list can be found in the publication by Gurwitt et al., 1992). Some symptoms seem interrelated in obvious or verifiable ways. For example, many people with or without Chronic Fatigue develop muscle aches and pains due to disturbed or otherwise inadequate sleep. As another example, at least some allergic reactions and sensitivities affect the central nervous system, which can cause muscle pain, fatigue, or both.

SEEKING HELP AND SUPPORT

Both before and after I was officially diagnosed by an M.D. as having Chronic Fatigue (only a few years ago), I sought help not only from the chiropractors, massage therapists, and acupuncturists mentioned earlier but also from various naturopaths, M.D. specialists from a wide range of fields, a physical therapist, and a physiatrist. I sought help both in Canada and in the United States. I even spent a year trying homeopathic drops described as created especially for me from India.

Gibson (2000) has found that the average sufferer of MCS sees 8.6 medical practitioners alone (not including alternative practitioners) and spends a mean of $5,784 a year on medical care and a mean of $34,783 over the course of their illness. Her data were gathered nearly ten years ago, so one wonders what comparable figures would be in today's costs. Furthermore, as Anderson (2000) notes, physicians often have little knowledge about or interest in symptoms that seriously hamper one's daily life if they are not "medically significant."

A common characteristic of CF/MCS is that few or no treatments of any kind are helpful in alleviating symptoms, and even those that initially yield a positive result soon stop working. Until a year ago, that was my experience. Various theories have been proposed to explain this lack of response to treatment, but little is known for certain. Another little-understood question is why different individuals develop somewhat different clusters of symptoms. Individual differences in pre-existing weaknesses of particular body systems may be responsible, but that has not been proven. Some people recover quickly, some gradually over many years, and others not at all. Once again, there is no proven explanation for this variability. What does seem clear is that some of us are like the canaries miners used to take down into coal mines. When the canaries died, it meant that there was too little oxygen at that level, so the miners knew to return closer to the earth's surface. Some humans seem to react sooner than others to the presence of toxic chemicals and even to dust and molds. A colleague of mine who said he had never been sick a day in his life began coughing badly the first day he worked in a sealed building and continued to cough every workday until soon after leaving the building. But based on my experience at OISE and on what I have seen happening to the people who have remained there, my personal impression is that most people are affected sooner or later if they stay long enough in that environment. In view of the wide range of individual differences in time between exposure to pathogens and the time one develops, or becomes aware of, symptoms, one possibility is that all exposed people are being harmed beginning with their first exposure but that in some people the harm takes longer to become apparent than in others. What does seem eminently sensible is to make a priority of widescale research and vigorous monitoring of indoor air quality and far more careful documentation of potentially dangerous levels of toxins than the economically and politically powerful chemical lobbies currently allow.

The variabilities related to Chronic Fatigue make it easy to claim that there is no such illness or that it is purely psychological, a product either of depression (allegedly producing the mistaken, pessimistic belief that one has all sorts of physical problems) or of a sick need for attention acquired through claiming to be ill (see, for instance, the troubling article by Abbey & Garfinkel, 1991). Fortunately, better work has recently been done in regard to this point, including that by Jason et al. (1997), who explain some of the errors in research methodology and interpretation of data that have led to the mistaken claim that CF is simply a psychiatric problem.

Based on my own experience, I can say with certainty that having a wide variety of physical problems, virtually none of which responds very much or at all to any kind of treatment, can be frustrating and depressing. Vivienne Anderson (2000) says of her experience with Chronic Fatigue that not pain but fatigue is the symptom she would most want to be rid of. When I was raising my children, feeling exhausted all the time made me quite certain that I was a bad mother: I couldn't run and play with them much, and had to hoard my energy by making meals and housekeeping as simple as possible and getting help from the children or other people whenever I could. Although I have been lucky that my mental energy has remained high most of the time, except when the physical exhaustion has become so profound that I have not been able to maintain concentration on a task, it is often physically painful or almost immediately exhausting to sit upright at my desk in order to write. But this very dramatic difference between the high level of my mental energy and the low level of my physical energy has proven immensely puzzling to people. This is exacerbated by the fact that the color in my cheeks makes me look very healthy, although sometimes my color is high because it is one manifestation of my chemical sensitivities. Furthermore, having lived with this condition for nearly two decades, I have spent an enormous amount of energy planning and rearranging my life. For instance, if I have to write a paper or testify in court or give a keynote address, I take great care to minimize everything else I have to do before and afterward, including cooking and shopping. As a consequence, what most other people see is only a woman with pink cheeks who seems in their view to do a lot of work (I seem to have been born, luckily, with the ability to write and to plan lectures pretty quickly) and doesn't seem tired.

If I had spent all these years giving people regular reports on my various symptoms, I doubt that I would have any friends left at all. So it's a Catch-22: informing people regularly about one's symptoms carries a huge risk of rejection, but trying one's best to cope and not complain and to enjoy life as much as possible makes it look as though there really is no problem, so people don't believe it when you come smack up against your limitations. Anderson (2000) writes that the need of the ill to "pass" for healthy contributes to the lack of discussion and therefore knowledge about chronic illness in the general population. She also writes that, because ill people are having to focus so much on surviving their illness that they do not write about it, the realities of their lives go unnoticed by social planners and even feminists.

It was ironic that I experienced one of my worst drops in physical energy as a result of a viral infection just as I was needing to write this paper. Viruses sometimes, but not always, precipitate my asthma-like condition, which is called Reactive Airways Syndrome (RAS). I raised a son who has asthma, so I associate breathing problems with audible wheezing. But I rarely have audible wheezing, even when my breathing is labored. Furthermore, I have never known anyone who has RAS, and I am not in regular contact with anyone who has Chronic Fatigue. So, after I had a fever of close to 102 degrees Fahrenheit, despite a subsequent week of coughing, I actually failed to notice the bronchospasms. Once I noticed that, even when I was not coughing, breathing was difficult, the spasms had probably been going on for a week, and that makes it harder to break the spasm. Furthermore, this condition means that one is not getting enough oxygen, which leads to great fatigue. Then, in an experience typical for people with CFS/MCS, because we tend to be highly drug-sensitive, I had the dilemma of how to stop the breathing problem. From past experience, I knew I could not use most puffers, because even when the active ingredients help me, I tend to have an adverse reaction to the propellants. I tried a nebulizer for a week; it helped my breathing moderately up to a point and then did not seem to help further, and I had some strange and disturbing negative effects from the medication which my physician said could not be caused by the medication but a woman pharmacist said would follow quite logically from the way this medication operates. I then tried an inhaled steroid, but it made me incredibly sleepy and also caused severe stomach pains. Again, my doctor says the latter is impossible, but it has happened every one of the three or four times I have taken steroids. So has skyrocketing weight gain, this time twelve pounds in one week. I used to be a journalist and always meet my deadlines, but this time I was frustrated to have to try to rush all the writing of this paper into the day before it was due. (I was glad to have a chance to revise this paper later on.) In such a situation, one fears being considered a slacker and feels frustrated about being unable to do what one formerly could do with ease.

Feeling pretty powerless and even ashamed can be very depressing. But I have long been aware that virtually *anything* can make me feel genuinely happy: talking with a friend or loved one, hearing a joke, stepping outside when the snow has just fallen or the weather is warm and clear. That is not the pattern of a person whose depression is causing her to have or to imagine having physical problems. But the presence of depression or other upsetting emotions in people with CF or MCS is understandable and leads easily to the conclusion that the physical problems are not real. I worry about how many people are misdiagnosed as having a primary depression and fruitlessly or even harmfully put on psychotropic medication or started on years of misguided psychotherapy.

CHRONIC FATIGUE AS A WOMEN'S ISSUE

Chronic Fatigue is in many ways a women's issue. For one thing, as Anderson (2000) writes, "The chronically sick are a neglected subset of the disabled. They are often overlooked, in part because the stereotypical public image of the person with a disability is of a young, healthy, athletic, paraplegic male, such as the celebrated wheelchair athlete Rick Hansen." Furthermore, some research suggests that one or more aspects of women's hormonal makeup may render us more susceptible than males to the simultaneous exposure to multiple chemicals. Then, too, women are far more likely than men to have the kinds of jobs that keep them for long hours in sealed buildings. This is partly because lower-paid, lower-status workers, such as secretaries and cleaning staff, are less likely to have the freedom to take work home with them, and many building-bound tasks such as library work are done mostly by female staff. Furthermore, at OISE in particular, as at many institutions, the feminist faculty, nearly all of whom were female, were far more likely than other faculty to be swamped with thesis supervision responsibilities. In academic and other institutions in general, students, employees, and coworkers are far more likely to turn to women than to men when they need advice or support in regard to personal problems (e.g., see Caplan, 1993), so that aspect of work life tends to keep women in the building more hours per day. Finally, even female faculty or students who could take work such as reading or writing tasks home with them often prefer to do their work in their offices because when they are home they are more likely than men to be shouldering the vast majority of household and childcare responsibilities (e.g., see Caplan, 2000). These various factors seemed to lead to the greater reporting of Chronic Fatigue and related symptoms by women than by men at OISE, and, as in so many situations, this increased the likelihood that the symptoms would be "explained" as hysterical, hormonally-related in an offensive sense, or examples of nasty, militant feminists' attempts to make trouble whenever they can.

I have not been surprised, therefore, although I have been saddened, when women colleagues have told me in confidence that they have CF but that I must never tell anyone that they do. Perhaps they fear not only being de-scribed as hysterical but also losing friends and relationships with family members who might accuse them of being picky, paranoid, or self-indulgent or of refusing to acknowledge their human limitations by cutting back on work (see Gibson, Cheavens, & Warren, 1998; Anderson, 2000). Let me tell you a typical story from my own experience. A dear friend and I met at a restaurant she suggested. I asked the woman who seated us for a non-smok-ing table. We sat down and began to look at the menus. Someone lit up a cigarette at the next table. I asked our server if she could request that the smoker put out the cigarette. She explained that our table was right next to the smoking section. I asked if we could move as far away as possible. My friend rolled her eyes. We moved. My friend suggested I order a particular dish, but I explained that, although it sounded delicious, I could not eat it because it contained oats. She suggested another one, and I had to say that dishes with coconut that comes from a can usually contain the preservative sodium bisul-fite, to which I have a terrible reaction. My friend exploded, "Oh Paula, for God's sake!" and rarely had time to get together with me after that. Anderson (2000) suggests that some people are unable to be around those who are ill because it makes them aware that they, too, could become ill. Chronic illness also may try the patience of family and friends; Cherie Register (1987) calls people with ongoing health problems the "interminably ill."

During most of the years that I have had CF, I did not know anyone else who definitely had it, so when I read Pamela Gibson's (Gibson et al., 1998; Gibson, 2000) reports of the frequency of such experiences of loss and rejection of people with MCS, I wept at seeing my life described on her pages. It was the first breakdown in the isolation I had felt. It is hard to be called names when one simply wants to feel better and is frustrated by lacking the stamina to complete work projects or even hold a job, to try to enjoy life despite frequent or unremitting pain, to try to be a good mother while constantly feeling exhausted.

THE REST OF MY STORY

The OISE administration's failure even to respond to my request for space in an unsealed building after my sabbatical year worried me. A labor lawyer advised me that their nonresponse was an attempt at "constructive dismissal." If I failed to resume teaching in the OISE building when my sabbatical ended, he said, the administration quite likely would stop my paychecks, and I would have to file a lawsuit against them and hope to win it. He said further that Sick Building Syndrome had not been litigated in Ontario, and so he could charge me tens of thousands of dollars and give me no better than 50-50 odds of winning. I asked him to negotiate a settlement for me, because the clear choice was between my job and my health. I received a settlement that turned out to be pitifully small in view of my learning over the past six years that staying out of sealed buildings and moving to a less polluted city would do little or nothing to alleviate my health problems. The symptoms, it seemed, were signs not of temporary illness but of damage. I did pay the lawyer a huge sum for negotiating the settlement. Not long after the settlement was signed, when I had reason to believe that someone in the OISE administration had gone against our settlement agreement by providing a negative recommendation when I was applying for an academic job, I asked the same lawyer to send a letter reminding them of the terms of the agreement. He refused to do so, on the grounds that he had taken on a client whose interests would conflict with mine. I considered his conduct to be ethically questionable, but frankly, I had no energy left to file a complaint against him. So I quietly accepted what he said and felt powerless. Despite applying for jobs for which I am well qualified or even overqualified, in the four years after I knew I was leaving OISE I never even made a short list. People have made comments directly to me that indicate that some people consider me to be a problem because the OISE building made me ill.

I filed for Workers' Compensation, was turned down, and have now been through every level of appeal but the final one, a process that has dragged on for years. My claim was refused on the grounds that:

- it is not clear whether my condition "is actually a clinical syndrome or a diagnostic entity on its own" (Does this make sense? I thought some diagnostic entities *were* clinical syndromes);
- the causes of the alleged syndrome are not clear (So that means it doesn't exist? When nonsmokers get lung cancer, does one deny that they have that illness?);

- the medical benefits of treatment provided by clinical ecologists were not clear (I had not claimed to have been much helped, just reported seeking treatment and requested reimbursement for that.);
- the American Medical Association does not recognize a valid diagnosis for my condition, and therefore there is no way to evaluate the nature or severity of my complaints.

SOME HELP AT LAST

In June of 1999, something made me check in with the Toronto naturopath whom I had not seen in years. I noted that it was now clear that my many health problems, for some of which she had recommended treatments in the past, constituted Chronic Fatigue. She had learned new things in recent years, and after doing some laboratory tests, she suggested that I take some combinations of a large number of homeopathic drops. My skepticism about still more treatment was overcome by the results. Within a few weeks, the feeling of tiredness at the back of my eyes left me for the first time in nearly twenty years. Sleep left me feeling rested. Mild to moderate exercise no longer wore me out. With few changes in what I ate (nothing that I hadn't tried several times over the years) and none in the amount, I became less reactive to a number of foods, became more physically resilient (e.g., too few hours of sleep no longer leads to a crash), and lost 23 pounds in 20 weeks. As mentioned, many problems remain, the most distressing being the intermittent breathing problems, and I continue to have many food and chemical allergies and sensitivities, among other symptoms. I still take and quite likely will always have to take large numbers of vitamins, minerals, enzymes, and other supplements. Currently, I take 26 pills every morning, 15 with lunch, 15 with dinner, and 14 at bedtime because I feel worse if I do not, and this amounts to a great deal of expense. To give one small example of the ongoing problems, an evening at the theatre can become an almost unbearable experience if I sit next to someone wearing perfume.

Today, I am enormously grateful to my naturopath, and I hope that I may gradually come to feel even better. However, even if I do not, I feel as though in many important ways I have my life back. I wish that all sufferers from these kinds of problems could say as much. I wish that I could tell you that my naturopath knows other practitioners who do the kind of work she does, but I have asked her to recommend people in other geographical areas, and she says that in all honesty she has not been able to find anyone who works in the ways she does. I do feel that all the years of subjection to mockery for refusing to give up hope, for constantly trying new things, for longing to feel better, were worth it because, had I given up, I would feel no better now. But for many of us, there are limits to how closely we shall ever approach what is called "normal" physical health, and this is especially distressing when we live in a culture in which, in the words of Roanne Thomas-Maclean (in press), "'Normal' is a quality to which one must return," to which one is expected and pressured to return.

I recommend Pamela Reed Gibson's careful, comprehensive, sensitive, and helpful work (Gibson, 2000; Gibson et al., 1996, 1998), as well as that of Lauerman (1997), Anderson (2000), and Thomas-Maclean (in press) for those of you whose stories sound at all like mine. I have also learned a great deal about the effects of chemical exposures from the Chemical Injury Information Network's monthly publication, "Our Toxic Times," which can be ordered at P.O. Box 301, White Sulphur Springs, Montana 59645-0301; phone (406) 547-2255; fax (406) 547-2455.

SUGGESTIONS FOR THERAPISTS

It is important for therapists to keep in mind the complexity of the issues related to Chronic Fatigue and similar disorders, and I have tried to illustrate some of these complexities here. They include the facts that:

- in any given person, the kinds of symptoms described in this paper may or may not have underlying physical causes such as CFS/MCS;
- researchers and clinicians are only beginning to understand the etiology of such illnesses as well as the variability in symptom pictures, the duration from exposure to problem-causing substances to the onset of noticeable symptoms, the duration of the illness, and the chances for full recovery;
- there is a paucity of practitioners who know much about these kinds of illnesses; and
- there is a paucity of effective treatments.

In spite of these complexities and uncertainties, there is a great deal that therapists can do to be helpful.

Therapists should remember that physical problems can be misinterpreted as psychologically-caused but also that psychological problems can be misinterpreted as physically-caused. It is especially tricky to identify causation when the physical problems are, or may be, part of a physical disorder that is not widely known to exist or is mistakenly regarded as psychological, as even tuberculosis was before the tubercle bacillus was discovered.

Therapists can keep in mind that people who have sought treatment from many professionals for physical problems may be not emotionally disturbed attention-seekers but rather people with genuine physical illness, even if they do not have concomitant abnormalities on such measures as blood tests or X rays.

Therapists can remember that people with these types of chronic health problems have often lost the support of loved ones, the ability to earn an income, even the ability to maintain concentration or to carry out many tasks of self-care.

Therapists can become informed about which local health practitioners know the most about little-understood physical health problems, perhaps even practitioners or laypeople who have such illness themselves, and which practitioners are most respectful toward those who struggle with these kinds of symptoms.

Therapists can be helpful in assisting the sufferer to:

- keep or regain trust in her own perceptions about her physical condition. Encouraging the patient to keep a journal of the timing of her symptoms and where she is when they arise can be useful in helping her ·to identify patterns and causal connections. Above all, encourage the patient to trust that she knows better than anyone else how she feels. Related to this, the patient should be encouraged to avoid as much as possible spending time in environments that cause their symptoms and/ or to investigate whether measures such as the use of ozone-producing air purifiers can help. Such purifiers have dramatically reduced my brain fog and headaches when I have had to spend time in sealed buildings, such as in libraries when doing research.
- maintain self-respect in the face of others' disbelief or rejection.

Therapists can familiarize themselves with the kinds of medical symptom histories described in this article and in the references listed at its end.

Therapists can encourage the patient to talk or otherwise communicate with other people who have had similar problems, such as making contacts through "Our Toxic Times" (mentioned above) or through the internet or local support groups.

ACKNOWLEDGMENTS

I am grateful to my parents, Tac and Jerry Caplan, for their support of all kinds always and especially for their wonderfully insightful and sensitive suggestions and comments about this paper. I am also grateful to Ellyn Kaschak for her great editorial wisdom and to Pamela Reed Gibson for her wonderful work and her assistance with this paper.

REFERENCES

Abbey, Susan, and Garfinkel, Paul. (1991). Neurasthenia and Chronic Fatigue Syndrome: The role of culture in the making of a diagnosis. *American Journal of Psychiatry 148*: 1638-1646.

Anderson, Vivienne. (2000). A will of its own: Experiencing the body in severe chronic illness. In Baukje Miedema, Janet Stoppard, & Vivienne Anderson (Eds.), *Women's Bodies/Women's Lives*. Toronto: Sumach Press.

Blank, Dennis M. (1998). What's in the office air? Workers smell trouble. *The New York Times*, Feb. 22, 1998, p. 11.

Caplan, Paula J. (2000). *The New Don't Blame Mother: Mending the Mother-Daughter Relationship*. New York: Routledge.

Caplan, Paula J. (1995). *They Say You're Crazy: How the World's Most Powerful Psychiatrists Decide Who's Normal.* Reading, MA: Addison-Wesley.

Caplan, Paula J. (1994). *The Myth of Women's Masochism*. Toronto: University of Toronto Press.

Caplan, Paula J. (1993). *Lifting a Ton of Feathers: A Woman's Guide to Surviving in the Academic World*. Toronto: University of Toronto Press.

Caplan, Paula J. (1992). Driving us crazy: How oppression damages women's mental health and what we can do about it. *Women & Therapy, 12* (5): 5-28.

Caplan, Paula J. (1991). How *do* they decide who is normal? The bizarre, but true, tale of the *DSM* process. *Canadian Psychology/Psychologie Canadienne, 32:* 162-170.

Caplan, Paula J., and Gans, Maureen. (1991). Is there empirical justification for the category of "Self-defeating Personality Disorder"? *Feminism and Psychology, 1:* 263-78.

Caplan, Paula J., McCurdy-Myers, Joan, and Gans, Maureen. (1992). Should "premenstrual syndrome" be called a psychiatry abnormality? *Feminism and Psychology, 2:* 27-44.

Duehring, Cindy. (1997). Objective injuries in Gulf War veterans echo MCS and implicate chemical synergy. *Our Toxic Times*. November, 13-17.

Gibson, Pamela Reed. (2000). *Multiple Chemical Sensitivity: A Survival Guide.* Oakland: New Harbinger Publications.

Gibson, Pamela Reed, Cheavens, Jennifer, and Warren, Margaret. (1998). Social support in persons with self-reported sensitivity to chemicals. *Research in Nursing and Health, 21*(2): 103-115.

Gibson, Pamela Reed, Cheavens, Jennifer, and Warren, Margaret. (1996). Multiple chemical sensitivity/environmental illness and life disruption. *Women & Therapy, 19*: 63-79.

Gurwitt, Alan, Barrett, Sharon, Brown, Sunnie, Butaney, Edna, Gorman, Bonnie, Kilgore, James, O'Grady, Erin, Potaznick, Walter, Saltzstein, Barbara, Sanford, Ann, Webster, Warnie, & Zimmer, Victoria. (1992). Chronic Fatigue Syndrome: A primer for physicians and allied health professionals. Waltham, MA: Massachusetts CFIDS Association (808 Main Street, Waltham, MA 02154).

Jason, Leonard, Richman, Judith, Friedberg, Fred, Wagner, Lynne, Taylor, Renee, & Jordan, Karen. (1997). Politics, science, and the emergence of a new disease: The case of Chronic Fatigue Syndrome. *American Psychologist, 52*(9): 973-83.

Lauerman, John F. (1997). The elusive diagnosis. *Harvard Magazine,* October, 19-22.

Pantony, Kaye-Lee, and Caplan, Paula J. (1991). Delusional Dominating Personality Disorder: A modest proposal for identifying some consequences of rigid masculine socialization. *Canadian Psychology/Psychologie Canadienne, 32*: 120-33.

Quinn, Christopher. (1997). What causes fibromyalgia? *Living with Fibromyalgia.* Sponsored by Rehabilitation Hospital of Rhode Island and Arthritis Foundation, Southern New England Chapter. December, pp. 1-4.

Register, Cherie. (1987). *Living with Chronic Illness: Days of Patience and Passion.* New York: Macmillan.

Thomas-Maclean, Roanne. (in press). Altered bodies/altered selves: Exploring women's accounts of illness experiences. In Baukje Miedema, Janet Stoppard, & Vivienne Anderson (Eds.), *Women's Bodies/Women's Lives.* Toronto: Sumach Press.

Fibromyalgia:
A Feminist Biopsychosocial Perspective

Mary Terrell White

Jeanne Parr Lemkau

Mark E. Clasen

SUMMARY. Fibromyalgia (FM) is a syndrome predominantly experienced by women and characterized by pain, fatigue, sleep disturbance, and multiple tender points at distinct locations on the body. Because of its prevalence and the common comorbidity of FM with depression and other conditions that prompt sufferers to seek psychological care, it is incumbent upon psychologists to be familiar with the syndrome, competent to provide assistance to afflicted individuals, and aware of the impact of gender politics on fibromyalgia sufferers. We present an overview of the diagnosis and treatment of fibromyalgia, a brief summary of etiological possibilities, and a discussion of the experience of illness among affected individuals. We conclude by exploring the social construction of the syndrome from a feminist perspective. *[Article copies available for a fee from The Haworth Document Delivery Service: 1-800-342-9678. E-mail address: <getinfo@haworthpressinc.com> Website: <http://www.Haworth Press.com> © 2001 by The Haworth Press, Inc. All rights reserved.]*

KEYWORDS. Fibromyalgia, fibrositis, chronic illness

The authors are each members of the faculty at Wright State University School of Medicine in Dayton, Ohio. Mary Terrell White, PhD, is Assistant Professor in the Department of Community Health; Jeanne Parr Lemkau, PhD, is Clinical Psychologist in the Department of Family Medicine, and Mark E. Clasen, MD, is Chair of the Department of Family Medicine.

Address correspondence to: Mary T. White, PhD, Department of Community Health, WSU-SOM, P.O. Box 927, Dayton, OH 45401-0927.

[Haworth co-indexing entry note]: "Fibromyalgia: A Feminist Biopsychosocial Perspective." White, Mary Terrell, Jeanne Parr Lemkau, and Mark E. Clasen. Co-published simultaneously in *Women & Therapy* (The Haworth Press, Inc.) Vol. 23, No. 1, 2001, pp. 45-58; and: *Minding the Body: Psychotherapy in Cases of Chronic and Life-Threatening Illness* (ed: Ellyn Kaschak) The Haworth Press, Inc., 2001, pp. 45-58. Single or multiple copies of this article are available for a fee from The Haworth Document Delivery Service [1-800-342-9678, 9:00 a.m. - 5:00 p.m. (EST). E-mail address: getinfo@haworthpressinc.com].

Fibromyalgia (FM) is a controversial disorder characterized by generalized pain and stiffness, fatigue, sleep disturbance, and multiple reproducible tender points at symmetrical locations on the body. Although the symptoms of the disorder have long been recognized as a source of suffering and help-seeking, especially among women, only recently has the condition been recognized by the medical community. Given the prevalence of the disorder in an aging population and the common comorbidity of FM and depression, it is important for psychologists to be familiar with the syndrome, competent to provide assistance to afflicted individuals, and aware of the impact of gender politics on fibromyalgia sufferers. To that end, we provide an overview of the diagnosis and treatment of fibromyalgia and several etiological possibilities under investigation. We follow this overview with a discussion of the illness as experienced by afflicted individuals, and conclude by considering the social construction of this disorder from a feminist perspective.

DEFINITION AND HISTORY

"Fibromyalgia" denotes a painful (algos) condition (ia) of the muscle (myo) fibers (fibro), a condition characterized by the presence of numerous painfully tender points symmetrically located on the body. Although muscle pain has been described in medical literature for centuries, tender points were first associated with disease in the early 1800s, when recognized as a symptom of rheumatism. At the turn of the century, the term "fibrositis" was coined to refer to general muscle pain thought to be caused by inflammation of muscle tissues. In the 1930s, a condition involving numerous specific, reproducible tender points was distinguished from both general muscle pain and "trigger points," which, when palpated, generate referred pain in other distant locations (Powers, 1993). In the 1960s, tender points were recognized as one of a cluster of symptoms that primarily appeared in women, along with muscle pain and stiffness, poor sleep, and headaches. With the exception of tender points, affected women were normal on physical examination. For this reason, tender points were identified as the hallmark feature of what was still called "fibrositis" (Smythe and Moldolfsky, 1977). The term "fibromyalgia" was subsequently introduced to replace "fibrositis" because no inflammation of muscle tissue had been demonstrated (Yunus, Masi, Calabro, Miller, Feigenbaum, 1981).

In 1990 the American College of Rheumatology endorsed classification criteria for the fibromyalgia syndrome (Wolfe, Smythe, Yunus, Bennett, Bombardier, Goldenberg et al., 1990). The disorder was subsequently recognized by the World Health Organization in 1992. Because no clear pathophysiological explanation of FM exists, the disorder is referred to as a syndrome rather than a disease.

Persons diagnosed with fibromyalgia commonly experience debilitating fatigue, chronic pain, and sleeplessness. These symptoms can disrupt performance, interpersonal relationships, the pursuit of personal goals, and tend to generate secondary reactions of anxiety and depression. Diagnosis is often elusive as symptoms vary widely, and relatively few physicians are familiar with the syndrome or competent to make a diagnosis. Clinicians and patients alike may initially minimize or dismiss complaints as transitory or psychosomatic. In some cases, negative gender stereotypes of women may support views of sufferers as hypochondriacs and malingerers.

Women who experience the ambiguous yet debilitating symptoms of fibromyalgia in a social context that evokes negative gender attributes are understandably stressed both during the period prior to diagnosis and subsequently, as they adjust to the realities of managing a chronic condition. For those women able and willing to seek psychological help, supportive psychotherapy can be a most helpful adjunct to medical care. A feminist psychological perspective on fibromyalgia is also useful in mental health consultations provided by psychologists and other mental health professions in primary care medical settings.

EPIDEMIOLOGY

The overall prevalence of FM in the general US population is estimated at between 0.7% and 6% (Clauw, 1995; Lorenzen, 1994; Wolfe, Ross, Anderson, Russell, & Hebert, 1995), with women being affected up to ten times more frequently than men (Lorenzen, 1994). Although FM can develop from childhood to old age, its prevalence seems to increase with age, with the highest prevalence occurring among women between ages 60 and 79 (Wolfe et al., 1995). Prevalence rises within medical clinic populations; some rheumatologists consider FM to be the predominant condition they see, especially in women under fifty (Bennett, 1995; Bennett, Smythe and Wolfe, 1992; Wolfe et al., 1995). The actual incidence of the disorder is difficult to establish as estimates vary depending on the criteria used for diagnosis and the population from which a study sample is drawn.

CLINICAL PRESENTATION

Persons afflicted with FM typically complain of muscle pain in the neck, shoulders, back, and pelvis. The pain is variously described as diffuse and stabbing, constant and intermittent, dull, exhausting, nagging, radiating, and/or spreading. Pain may be exacerbated with fatigue, stress or changes in weather, and alleviated with hot baths, heating pads, warm weather, mild exercise, and/or rest (Powers, 1993). Muscle pain and stiffness are often accompanied by disturbed and non-restorative sleep. FM sufferers are often sedentary and deconditioned, although whether this is a cause or effect of their symptoms is unclear.

FM is not life-threatening. However, it often develops in people previously diagnosed with potentially serious connective tissue diseases, such as rheumatoid arthritis, Sjogren's disease, or lupus. Several long term studies of FM sufferers found chronic but nonprogressive symptoms to be the rule, with waxing and waning of symptoms from day to day. Many individuals report substantial improvement in symptoms over time, although whether this reflects a true physiological change or improved adaptation to the condition is difficult to determine (Bennett, 1995). One prospective long-term study found symptoms to last, on average, at least 15 years after the onset of illness (Kennedy and Felson, 1996). Others note a more positive prognosis with early diagnosis and appropriate medical management (Wallace, 1997).

The unique feature of FM is the presence of unusual tenderness at anatomically reproducible, symmetric locations which are only slightly tender in normal persons. Although FM sufferers typically report generalized pain, they may be unaware of the extreme sensitivity of these specific points prior to palpation by the physician. Unless there is comorbid disease, physical examination beyond the tender point exam is typically normal, with negative laboratory and radiologic studies. An exception is sleep lab studies, which have revealed an alpha-delta sleep disturbance which is not specific to FM (Clauw, 1995; Powers, 1993). Other symptoms commonly associated with FM but not essential to the diagnosis include tension headaches, dizziness, cold sensitivity, fluid retention, concentration difficulties, a subjective sense of swelling, and feelings of numbness and tingling. Associated medical conditions may include irritable bowel or bladder syndromes, transmandibular joint pain (TMJ), dysmenorrhea, migraine headaches, depression, restless leg syndrome, and a variety of connective tissue diseases. Chronic fatigue syndrome may co-occur; in fact, many believe CFS and FM to be different manifestations of the same disease spectrum, with fatigue symptoms predominating in CFS and pain symptoms in FM (Clauw, 1995). The similarities between the two, as well as multiple chemical sensitivity, has led to the suggestion that diagnoses may depend more on the treating physician's specialty area than the actual course of illness (Buchwald and Garrity, 1994).

DIAGNOSIS

The American College of Rheumatology Criteria for the classification of FM includes a history of widespread pain of at least three months duration and pain on digital palpation of a minimum of 11 of 18 specific tender points

(Wolfe et al., 1990). The cardinal diagnostic feature of the disorder is tenderness at these anatomically reproducible sites. However, the diagnostic criteria have generated criticism on several grounds. The criteria were established from a study of people previously diagnosed with fibromyalgia. Because the majority of these persons exhibited tender points, it was concluded that the presence of tender points could be used to identify persons with FM. This reasoning has been criticized as circular (Bohr, 1995; Cohen and Quintner, 1993; Raspe and Croft, 1995); moreover, the criteria are unclear as to how the subjective experience of pain is to be measured, and whether a patient's history of pain must be constant or intermittent. Finally, because the criteria fail to indicate any pathophysiological cause, it cannot be assumed that FM is a single condition.

Despite these shortcomings, the establishment of diagnostic criteria for FM serves several useful functions. By providing a means of identifying and classifying persons suffering from a recognizable set of symptoms, the criteria draw attention to the prevalence of the disorder and provide an impetus for research. Most importantly, the criteria provide medical legitimacy for persons suffering from FM, enhancing their ability to command serious medical attention, obtain insurance coverage, and receive consideration for disability compensation.

Finally, the ACR criteria provide a basis for distinguishing FM from related disorders. The differential diagnosis is large and includes myofascial pain syndrome, chronic fatigue, malignancy, osteoarthritis, rheumatoid arthritis, polymyalgia rheumatica, and other connective tissue diseases such as systemic lupus erythematosus, polymyositis, and ALS. Typically, alternative explanations are ruled out by physical, laboratory, and/or X ray exams. Because FM symptoms may coexist with or represent the prodromal phase of some of these disorders, ongoing medical monitoring is appropriate.

ETIOLOGY

The symptoms characteristic of FM suggest musculoskelatal, neuroendocrinological, and psychiatric origins, however, the etiology of fibromyalgia is currently unknown. Research efforts have focused on changes in the muscular and circulatory systems, serotonin metabolism and central nervous system abnormalities, sleep disturbance, genetics, and psychiatric causes, with few significant and/or replicated findings.

Given that FM is characterized by pain in peripheral tissues, some change in muscle function or tissue morphology might be expected. However, extensive examination of muscle function and tissue morphology is inconclusive. Persons with FM are often aerobically unfit due to the pain and exhaustion that accompany exercise, thus some abnormalities in strength, endurance, and blood flow may be attributable to deconditioning rather than causally contributing to the syndrome (Bennett and Jacobsen, 1994; Henriksson, 1994; Yunus, 1994).

Because peripheral tissue sensitivity is common for persons with FM, a central mechanism has been sought to account for the syndrome. Pain may be exacerbated due to a hyperreactivity to normal sensations or to a reduction in the descending inhibitory pain pathways. According to one hypothesis, FM may be caused by a deficiency in serotonin, a neurotransmitter that inhibits pain in the descending pathway and promotes stage four sleep. Low plasma tryptophan, a precursor of serotonin, as well as low levels of serotonin, have been found in persons with FM (Neeck and Reidel, 1994), suggesting that abnormal serotonin metabolism may be implicated as either a cause or effect of FM.

Studies of family members indicate a higher than expected incidence of FM and related disorders (Clauw, 1995), raising the possibility of a genetic component. The data thus far are inconclusive, suggesting a polygenic or multifactorial pattern of inheritance, in which genetic factors are modified by gender, psychosocial, and environmental variables.

Yeast infections have also been posited as a possible contributor to FM, chronic fatigue, and other conditions that affect the immune system (Crook, 1995). Although this position currently finds little support in the mainstream medical literature, it suggests yet another possible causal mechanism.

Whenever a medical condition is poorly understood, psychiatric explanations abound, especially when the sufferers are preponderantly women. Studies suggest that 30% of FM patients have a psychiatric diagnosis, most often depression. However, since 70% of persons with FM do not suffer from a psychiatric disorder, the condition cannot be considered primarily psychiatric in nature (Bennett, 1995). Despite the absence of a consistent psychological profile of persons suffering from FM, case-controlled studies indicate that FM sufferers have higher rates of pre-morbid sexual and physical abuse, eating disorders, and drug abuse, suggesting that emotional trauma may be a predisposing factor (Powers, 1993).

Stress certainly seems to be correlated with both FM and typical concurrent disorders (such as TMJ or irritable bowel syndrome), but whether stress is a cause or an effect of FM is not clear. In one study, one third of the cases of FM seem to be precipitated by emotional or physical trauma (Greenfield et al., 1992). Another study found that patients with FM suffered more pain and life stress, and had more sleep disturbance than controls (Uveges et al., 1990). In a review of the psychological studies of FM using a variety of instruments, Yunus (1994) found that stress, as measured on an adjusted Hassles Scale, is more significant among those with FM than rheumatoid arthritis (Dailey et al., 1990). Anxiety is not significantly elevated in persons with FM compared with persons with rheumatoid arthritis, but depression may be more prevalent, supporting the view that depression is not caused exclusively by pain (Hawley and Wolfe, 1993). Regardless of whether it is a cause or effect, the psychological factors that accompany FM require as much recognition and treatment as the physical manifestations.

In summary, available research suggests that fibromyalgia is probably not attributable to a single cause and it may not be a single disorder. Rather, it appears that biological, psychological, and social factors may contribute synergistically to the development and perpetuation of the syndrome.

TREATMENT

A variety of interventions from across the biopsychosocial range have been found to be helpful to at least some FM sufferers. The most common treatments involve patient education and reassurance, drugs, aerobic exercise, and stress management. Multiple interventions are generally more helpful than any single treatment modality, hence a treatment team consisting of a primary care physician, a mental health professional, and a physical and/or occupational therapist is often required.

Patient education and reassurance are aimed toward enhancing patient involvement in other aspects of treatment and ameliorating secondary anxiety and depression. Because the symptoms of FM can be so varied and severe, many patients benefit from reassurance that they do not have a progressive or life-threatening disease, and support as they make necessary changes in their lives and grieve their losses.

Pharmacological treatments are directed at improving sleep, relaxing painful muscles, and decreasing pain, and may include tricyclic antidepressants, specific serotonin reuptake inhibitors (SSRIs), muscle relaxants, and pain medications. Low doses of antidepressants often improve sleep and lessen pain. Some trial and error is the norm.

Graded exercise to increase aerobic fitness and improve sleep tends to decrease symptoms. Women who are not incapacitated by pain usually find that regular, light exercise, such as walking, significantly improves their functioning. Overexertion can exacerbate symptoms, challenging the patient to find the optimum balance between exercise and rest. Massage and heat often alleviate symptoms of pain and tenderness.

Stress management is useful for controlling symptoms and minimizing secondary effects of the disorder. As with any chronic illness, supportive psychotherapy, grief work, and psychological treatment of comorbid conditions may be indicated. The "medical crisis counseling" approach, outlined by Pollin (1995) focusing on such issues as self-image, dependency, and fears of abandonment, provides a useful conceptual model for the psychological treatment of those who face unpredictable but not life-threatening chronic illnesses.

As with any chronic illness, a strong working alliance between the patient and her health care team is crucial. Patients appreciate professionals who validate their experiences of illness and thereby encourage them to become knowledgeable about the syndrome and expert in managing their symptoms.

THE PATIENT'S EXPERIENCE

Knowledge of typical experiences of patients with FM should inform psychological treatment. Those affected with FM face numerous challenges for which they are rarely prepared. Many of these challenges have been described in qualitative studies of FM sufferers in Scandinavia and the United States (Henriksson, 1995a, 1995b; Henriksson and Burkhardt, 1996).

Perhaps the most problematic aspect of this illness is the discrepancy between the patient's experience of pain and suffering and the absence of both objective physical findings and a biomedical explanation. That sufferers typically look healthy increases the risk that they will be dismissed or inappropriately treated within the medical system. This discrepancy may also be confusing to others within a woman's social network, who may respond with skepticism to someone who looks healthy but claims to be ill. Some women report negative reactions at work when they cannot do simple lifting or other chores that would be expected of a healthy person. Family and friends may be frightened by the illness and withdraw. Patients need ongoing support to help nurture and maintain social and family relationships stressed by the illness.

The period between when someone notices symptoms and receives an accurate diagnosis may be lengthy—in one study, the average was 6.7 years (Liller, 1994). During this time a woman may be sent from one specialist to another without receiving either an accurate diagnosis or acknowledgment that something is wrong (Henriksson, 1995a). Such dismissal undermines their confidence in their own knowledge, exacerbates anger and frustration, and adds to the psychological burden of the disorder.

When a diagnosis of fibromyalgia is finally made and explained to a patient, her reaction is often one of profound relief. Nevertheless, most FM sufferers must significantly alter their daily activities in order to manage their symptoms and adjust to the psychological impact of their illness (Henriksson, 1995b). The greatest physical discomfort is often in the morning, when muscle stiffness, pain, and cognitive difficulties are at their worst, and necessitate extra time and effort to get up and moving. Because symptoms change from day to day, it may be impossible to anticipate accurately what one will be able to manage at any given time. Motor abilities may become seriously limited, with the result that routine tasks such as doing laundry or cooking may require extra planning, effort, and time. Diminished physical abilities may also require sufferers to curtail activities that have been meaningful sources of pleasure and self-esteem.

Women report adopting various coping strategies to deal with the demands of their homes and work environments. Straightforward tactics include asking others for help and giving more attention to body mechanics, organization, and rest. Whether a task is employment related, a domestic chore, or recreational, women report fatigue after about 20-30 minutes, necessitating short breaks. Mental attention may also be difficult to maintain. Adapting to these limitations requires women to be flexible, self-disciplined, willing to relinquish control and depend on others. These changes are especially problematic for women whose identity and self-esteem are predicated on high independent accomplishment.

In adapting to chronic illness, FM sufferers must face the reality that they can no longer count on being who they imagined themselves to be or hoped to become. The losses of both bodily integrity and a secure and predictable future are inevitably accompanied by frustration, anger, and grief, reactions which call for skilled and compassionate counseling.

Some women resist making changes, trying to maintain their former activities despite the pain and fatigue. Some adapt and move on to new lives with different possibilities and goals. And some succumb to varying degrees of depression, social withdrawal, and invalidism. However, the vast majority of FM sufferers are not incapacitated by their illness. By budgeting time and energy, paying attention to activity levels and body mechanics, complying with medical and psychological treatments to ameliorate symptoms, and to a certain extent simply disregarding pain, women can learn to live with FM, although managing their lives may require an extra effort of will.

Given the complex and ambiguous etiology of fibromyalgia, the losses and adaptations involved, and the sometimes unsympathetic medical response, psychotherapists who understand the biopsychosocial dimensions of the syndrome can be immensely helpful to affected women adjusting to the realities of chronic illness. Effective roles for the therapist include patient education, support, advocacy, and empowerment. Therapists can help their clients locate compassionate and knowledgeable medical care and work collaboratively with women and their physicians. The affirmation of a woman's life experience, including her bodily experience, is especially important during illness, and a helpful antidote to the objectification she is likely to experience within the medical system. Ultimately, the aim of psychotherapy is to facilitate a woman's optimal functioning as she adapts her personality and family and work responsibilities to the realities of a chronic and unpredictable illness.

THE SYNDROME IN SOCIETY: A FEMINIST PERSPECTIVE

Any description of disease or illness is influenced by the social and cultural context in which it arises. The preceding discussion of fibromyalgia has presented certain truths about the condition from the perspectives of clinical medicine and affected patients living in contemporary Western societies. Each of these perspectives is both illuminating and limited, as each reflects certain ways of perceiving and interpreting experience while neglecting others. A third, feminist, perspective offers additional insights into how the FM syndrome and the women who suffer from it are interpreted within medicine and society.

One of the most important contributions of feminist philosophy in recent years has been its critique of the epistemological assumptions of the scientific method. Contemporary clinical medicine is the product of modern science, the findings of which are commonly considered to be objective, universally valid, and authoritative. Nonetheless, science is not value-neutral. In medicine, the ways in which diseases are defined, explained, and experienced as illness are shaped by the prevailing medical model and dominant values of a particular society at a given historical moment. For example, Abbey and Garfinkel (1991) describe how in the late nineteenth century, the causal hypotheses proffered for neurasthenia focused on electricity, conservation of energy, reflex action, and evolution and heredity, each of which was a preoccupation of the scientific community at that time. Similarly, in the heyday of infectious disease control in the mid-twentieth century, causal explanations for chronic fatigue were sought first in viruses, and subsequently, as medical attention shifted to AIDS and environmental toxins, in immunology and allergies. Given the bias toward "fashionable" explanations, one must question why certain causal factors for FM have been explored and others have not.

Part of the answer lies in the values reflected in medical practice. The contemporary medical model is grounded in a scientific method based on values of objectivity, value-neutrality, and generalizability. However, in recent decades, feminist philosophers of science have suggested that this scientific method represents only one view of reality, one that excludes other important sources of knowledge. They describe the scientific method as a "male" form of epistemology, derived from studies in physics, and characterized by reductionistic, deductive thinking. A feminist epistemology, alternatively, values subjective experience, personal narratives, and contextual details. In this view, meaning is found through feelings and emotions; through connection, not detachment (Code, 1991). For women suffering from FM, the subjective realities of pain and fatigue govern their daily lives. But because subjective knowledge is personal, not universalizable, it is not considered acceptable evidence for "hard" science.

This distinction between the scientific and feminist epistemologies raises several important questions. If patients complain of pain and fatigue for which physicians can find no pathophysiological cause or evidence, whose knowledge is authoritative–that of the physician or the patient? In the absence of physical findings, people afflicted with FM have been accused of fabricating pain for secondary gain, or of merely manifesting psychological problems. How aggressively will biomedical aspects of the disorder be pursued if women's subjective complaints of pain and fatigue are trivialized or assumed to be psychological in origin? More problematic is the question of whether the contemporary medical model limits a clinician's diagnostic alternatives. This condition does not seem to be attributable to any single mechanism, but may result from multiple biological, psychological, and social causes. Is our current medical model capable of embracing integrative, as opposed to reductionistic, thinking? What might a feminist medical model look like?

In keeping with feminists' emphasis on contextual analysis, a feminist medical model would at minimum be sensitive to the political context in which illness is experienced and defined. FM is a controversial disorder in part because of the historical association of similar types of disease with negative stereotypes of women. Originating in the 19th century as hysteria and neurasthenia, FM has been described as the latest manifestation of a psychiatric disorder in a long trajectory of related illnesses that has included neuromyasthenia, Epstein-Barr virus, and chronic fatigue. Women in the nineteenth century have been interpreted as reacting to overly restrictive domestic roles; conversely, contemporary women with FM or chronic fatigue have been charged with trying to avoid excessive demands of work and family (Shorter, 1992). Either way, women are construed as evading responsibility, being psychologically weak, and unable to meet the cultural expectations of their gender. For this reason, and because of the persistent stigma associated with mental illness, many contemporary women with FM resist the suggestion that their illnesses might have a psychological component.

A feminist interpretation of FM thus may also contain limitations. While women's concerns that certain diagnoses may lead to negative gender stereotyping are historically justified, to deny for this reason that psychosocial factors may play an important role in FM is to impose yet another level of bias on medical inquiry. Whether a medical model or a political ideology, rigid adherence to either may inhibit broad-ranging consideration of diverse causal factors. Instead of trying to find a causal explanation that corresponds to our current scientific and social priorities, it is essential to be open-minded, even to "unfashionable" possibilities. For example, psychosocial factors previously identified within feminist psychology and demonstrated to relate to morbidity and mortality for other health disorders could be considered in relation to the preponderance of women among fibromyalgia sufferers. These factors include women's disadvantaged social position, the prevalence of physical and psychological trauma in women's lives, and the different social and cultural expectations and pressures faced by women and men.

FM thus presents many challenges. The challenge for patients is to learn to acknowledge and cope with painful, persistent, and debilitating symptoms. The challenge for psychotherapists is to validate their patients' experience of illness and explore contributing or complicating psychological factors, without insisting on or denying the possibility of a biomedical explanation. The challenge for physicians and researchers is to give adequate attention to an expanding range of possible biomedical and psychosocial factors without stigmatizing women in the process. In short, if this illness is to be understood and successfully treated, we must be willing to examine our assumptions, to think broadly and deeply about multiple, interactive contributors to illness, and to be open to what we discover.

REFERENCES

Abbey, S.E., & Garfinkel, P.E. (1991). Neurasthenia and chronic fatigue syndrome: The role of culture in the making of a diagnosis. *American Journal of Psychiatry, 148*:1638-1646.

Bennett, R.M. (1995). Fibromyalgia: The commonest cause of widespread pain. *Comprehensive Therapy, 21*:269-275.

Bennett, R.M., & Jacobsen, S. (1994). Muscle function and origin of pain in fibromyalgia. *Baillieres Clinical Rheumatology, 8*:721-746.

Bennett, R.M., Smythe, H.A., & Wolfe, F. (1992, March 15). Recognizing fibromyalgia. *Patient Care*, 211-228.

Bohr, T.W. (1995). Fibromyalgia syndrome and myofascial pain syndrome: Do they exist? *Neurologic Clinics, 13*:365-384.

Buchwald, D., & Garrity, D. (1994). Comparison of patients with chronic fatigue syndrome, fibromyalgia, and multiple chemical sensitivities. *Archives of Internal Medicine, 154*:2049-2053.

Clauw, D.J. (1995). The pathogenesis of chronic pain and fatigue syndromes, with special reference to fibromyalgia. *Medical Hypotheses, 44*:369-378.

Code, L. (1991). *What Can She know? Feminist Theory and the Construction of Knowledge.* Ithaca: Cornell University Press.

Cohen, M.L., & Quintner, J.L. (1993). Fibromyalgia syndrome: A problem of tautology. *The Lancet, 342*:906-909.

Crook, W.G. (1995). *The Yeast Connection and the Woman.* Jackson: Professional Books, Inc.

Dailey, P.A., Bishop, G.D., Russell, I.J., & Fletcher, E.M. (1990). Psychological stress and the fibrositis/fibromyalgia syndrome. *Journal of Rheumatology, 17*:1380-1385.

Greenfield, S., Fitzcharles, M.A., & Esdaile, J.M. (1992). Reactive fibromyalgia syndrome. *Arthritis & Rheumatism, 35*:678-681.

Hawley, D.J., & Wolfe, F. (1993). Depression is not more common in rheumatoid arthritis: A 10-year longitudinal study of 6153 patients with rheumatic disease. *Journal of Rheumatology, 20*:2025-2031.

Henriksson, C., & Burckhardt, C. (1996). Impact of fibromyalgia on everyday life: A study of women in the USA and Sweden. *Disability and Rehabilitation, 18*:241-248.

Henriksson, C.M. (1995a). Living with continuous muscular pain–Patient perspectives. Part I: Encounters and consequences. *Scandinavian Journal of Caring Sciences, 9*:67-76.

Henriksson, C.M. (1995b). Living with continuous muscular pain–Patient perspectives. Part II: Strategies for daily life. *Scandinavian Journal of Caring Sciences, 9*:77-86.

Henriksson, K.G. (1994). Chronic muscular pain: Aetiology and pathogenesis. *Balliere's Clinical Rheumatology, 8*:703-719.

Kennedy, M., & Felson, D.T. (1996). A prospective long-term study of fibromyalgia syndrome. *Arthritis & Rheumatism, 39*:682-685.

Liller, T.K. (1994). *Expanding Horizons: An Exploration of Fibromyalgia Syndrome.* Fibromyalgia Association of Greater Washington, Inc.

Lorenzen, D. (1994). Fibromyalgia: A clinical challenge. *Journal of Internal Medicine, 235*:199-203.

Neeck, G., & Riedel, W. (1994). Neuromediator and hormonal perturbations in fibromyalgia syndrome: Results of chronic stress? *Balliere's Clinical Rheumatology, 8*:763-775.

Pollin, I. (1995). *Medical Crisis Counseling: Short-Term Therapy for Long-Term Illness.* New York: Norton.

Powers, R. (1993). Fibromyalgia: An age old malady begging for respect. *Journal of General Internal Medicine, 8*:93-105.

Raspe, H., & Croft, P. (1995). Fibromyalgia. *Balliere's Clinical Rheumatology, 9*:599-614.

Shorter, E. (1992). *From Paralysis to Fatigue: A History of Psychosomatic Illness in the Modern Era.* New York: The Free Press.

Smythe, H.A., & Moldolfsky, H. (1977). Two contributions to understanding of the "fibrositis" syndrome. *Bulletin on the Rheumatic Diseases, 28*:928-931.

Uveges, J.M., Parker, J.C., Smarr, K.L., McGowan, J.F., Lyon, M.G., Irvin, W.S. et al. (1990). Psychological symptoms in primary fibromyalgia syndrome: Relationship to pain, life stress, and sleep disturbance. *Arthritis & Rheumatism, 33*:1279-83.

Wallace, D.J. (1997). The fibromaylgia syndrome. *Annals of Medicine, 29*:9-21.

Wolfe, F., Ross, K., Anderson, J., Russell, I.J., & Hebert, L. (1995). The prevalence and characteristics of fibromyalgia in the general population. *Arthritis & Rheumatism, 38*:19-28.

Wolfe, F., Smythe, H.A., Yunus, M.B., Bennett, R.M., Bombardier, C., Goldenberg, D.L. et al. (1990). The American College of Rheumatology 1990 criteria for the classification of fibromyalgia: Report of the Multicenter Criteria Committee. *Arthritis & Rheumatism, 33*:160-172.

Yunus, M.B. (1994). Psychological aspects of fibromyalgia syndrome: A component of the dysfunctional spectrum syndrome. *Balliere's Clinical Rheumatology, 8*:811-837.

Yunus, M.B., Masi, A.R., Calabro, J.J., Miller, K.A., & Feigenbaum, S.L. (1981). Primary fibromyalgia (fibrositis). Clinical study of 50 patients with matched controls. *Seminars in Arthritis and Rheumatism, 11*:151-171.

Battling Injury and Chronic Illness
in a Managed Care World:
A Case History

Judy R. Lerner
Maureen Reid-Cunningham

SUMMARY. This article will chronicle Judy R. Lerner's experiences with a serious injury and the exacerbation of a chronic illness, ensuing disability and the difficulty she had accessing disability and health care benefits through her employer's managed care plan. It will demonstrate how therapy affected her ability to deal with adversity and to mold a new life for herself. In particular, it will reveal the importance of her relationship with her therapist, which was based on relational theory, and the influence that the therapist's disclosure of her own chronic illness had on the course of the therapy. *[Article copies available for a fee from The Haworth Document Delivery Service: 1-800-342-9678. E-mail address: <getinfo@haworthpressinc.com> Website: <http://www.HaworthPress.com> © 2001 by The Haworth Press, Inc. All rights reserved.]*

Judy R. Lerner spent nearly 20 years as a consultant in human resources communication, helping major companies communicate key corporate issues and also their benefit programs. Address correspondence to: 5009 Alcove Avenue, Sherman Village, CA 91607 (E-mail: JudyLerne@aol.com).

Maureen Reid-Cunningham, LICSW, BCD, is a clinical social worker with over 25 years' experience in the human services field. She currently has a private practice in Cambridge, Massachusetts, and has worked with many women who live with chronic illness. Address correspondence to: 10 Harrington Road, Cambridge, MA 02140 (E-mail: maureenrc@compuserve.com).

[Haworth co-indexing entry note]: "Battling Injury and Chronic Illness in a Managed Care World: A Case History." Lerner, Judy R. and Maureen Reid-Cunningham. Co-published simultaneously in *Women & Therapy* (The Haworth Press, Inc.) Vol. 23, No. 1, 2001, pp. 59-74; and: *Minding the Body: Psychotherapy in Cases of Chronic and Life-Threatening Illness* (ed: Ellyn Kaschak) The Haworth Press, Inc., 2001, pp. 59-74. Single or multiple copies of this article are available for a fee from The Haworth Document Delivery Service [1-800-342-9678, 9:00 a.m. - 5:00 p.m. (EST). E-mail address: getinfo@haworthpressinc.com].

KEYWORDS. Chronic illness, disability, health care benefits, relational theory, managed care, disclosure

On June 21, 1996, Judy R. Lerner's life changed forever. A successful
consultant who traveled the world working upwards of 90 hours a week, she
fell down a flight of stairs, sustained multiple fractures of her right leg and
her left foot, underwent emergency surgery, spent a week hospitalized, then
returned home to recover, confined alone with casts on both legs to her
third-floor bedroom. From the beginning, she battled not only her injury and
loss of mobility, but also difficulty obtaining health and disability benefits
from her managed health care plan and her employer, who sponsored the
plan. As a result of her accident and an unsuccessful attempt to return to work
with no accommodations for her weakened state, Lerner suffered a "flare"
(exacerbation) of her chronic illness, fibromyalgia,[1] and was forced to take a
short-term disability leave from work.

She never recovered from her illness, applied for long-term disability
benefits under her employer's plan, and filed suit for the benefits denied her.[2]
She remains to this day out of work, collecting Social Security disability
benefits.

Lerner's saga took her from successful overachiever in the corporate
world, never satisfied with less than perfection, to non-working woman who
discovered a different personal identity, a new strength and a commitment to
advocate for other patients less able to do battle for themselves. In the course
of her therapy, she came to terms with old family issues, new personal values,
redefined relationships and a new sense of purpose.

This article will chronicle Lerner's experiences and the effects of her therapy. It will show how therapy affected her ability to deal with adversity and to
mold a new life for herself. In particular, it will reveal the importance of her
relationship with her therapist and the influence her therapist's own chronic
illness had on the process of the therapy.

Throughout, the authors will summarize the events as they unfold. Then,
each one, first Lerner as the patient, then Reid-Cunningham as the therapist,
will provide personal perspectives and observations.

THE ACCIDENT
AND THE BEGINNING OF THE BENEFIT BATTLES

On June 21, 1996, Lerner fell down the stairs at her townhouse in Cambridge, Massachusetts. With three breaks in her right leg and a broken left
foot, she emerged from emergency surgery with casts on both legs and no
mobility. After three days in the hospital, she was transferred to a rehabilitation hospital that specialized in severe disability.

LERNER: It took a while for the magnitude of my injury and my situation to hit. Just hours after coming out of anesthesia, I wanted a phone to check voice mails at the office and return business phone calls. But when I arrived at the rehabilitation hospital three days later, a sinking feeling overwhelmed me. Suddenly, I was surrounded by people in various states of severe disability; I hadn't yet concluded that I, too, was disabled. Throughout my life, the sight of blood or disfigurement had made me queasy, so I knew I was in for a bumpy ride.

I immediately began to fight back. I told the rehabilitation hospital that I wanted to complete a full evaluation of my physical capabilities and some basic training in how to take care of myself with casts on both legs as quickly as possible. Then I talked to my case manager at the managed care plan[3] and stated that I wanted to be discharged home for the remainder of my recovery.

That's when the fight began. My case manager said my request didn't fit the guidelines. I replied (after nearly 20 years as a benefits expert) that care at home would cost no more, and probably less, than inpatient care. It took several days to work through the bureaucracy and get released with round-the-clock home health aide care.

THE RETURN HOME AND THE BEGINNING OF THERAPY

A week after the accident, Lerner returned home. She had 24-hour home health care and daily at-home physical therapy sessions. A week after returning home, Lerner heard that her managed care plan might cut off home health care, in spite of the fact she had casts on both legs, was unable even to get out of bed unassisted, and lived in a three-story townhouse. Lerner sought help from the Employee Assistance Program (EAP) provided through work. The EAP contacted Maureen Reid-Cunningham, who started therapy with Lerner within two days.

LERNER: The accident had been bad enough. Then I had to undergo a mindless battle with my managed care company just to be sent home, even though home care would cost less. And little did I know the war was just beginning.

Just a week after returning home, my physical therapist "leaked" the news that the managed care plan might cut off home care. I flew into a panic. I could barely get onto the wheel chair unassisted. To get onto the porta-potty beside my bed or roll via wheel chair to the bathroom sink for sponge baths required the help of a home health aide. Confined to bed on the third floor, I couldn't handle medical, sanitation, or feeding needs.

Calling the EAP, I explained my situation. The psychologist on the other end of the phone suggested a therapist to help not only with post-injury trauma, but also as an advocate to help do battle, in other words, a social worker. I agreed and added, "But there's one more glitch. Since I can't move, can you find someone who can make house calls?" Maureen appeared at my bedside only two days later.

Maureen heard my story and focused on my immediate concern: the cutoff of home health care. She took notes on relevant names and phone numbers and promised to make calls to my doctors, my health care plan, and my employer, if necessary. I was no longer alone.

Thanks to Maureen's efforts, we got a reprieve. It would be almost another month before home health care benefits were, in fact, terminated.

REID-CUNNINGHAM: The severity of the external stressors affecting Judy was apparent from the beginning. Cutting off home care presented a threat to her health and safety. I acted both as advocate and therapist to resolve the situation, as well as to address Judy's fear and isolation. Attending to Judy's basic needs helped to establish my credibility and supported my promise to work with her on the issues important to her.

I was impressed with Judy's intelligence and wry wit. At once angry, terrified and articulate, she felt her very survival was being threatened. The depth of her pain appeared early in our relationship; the causes would be revealed as therapy progressed. Our connection[4] became one of the few things Judy could depend upon as her physical condition worsened and her relationships with her employer and co-workers deteriorated.

Initially I planned to see Judy up to three times (as an EAP provider) to assess her needs and stabilize the situation and make a referral to another therapist if continuing services were necessary. By our second session, however, Judy reported feeling strongly that she wanted to work with me on an ongoing basis. After obtaining authorization from the EAP company, I agreed to continue our work.

Several factors contributed to the rapid development of the therapeutic relationship. I provided assistance with concrete services and listened to her in a way that was new and comforting to her. We also shared the bond of invisible chronic illness.

The decision to disclose an illness to a client is complicated. It is essential for the therapist to be clear that the disclosure will serve the client and the development of the relationship rather than meeting the therapist's needs. Given the critical situation Judy faced, it was necessary to establish a strong alliance quickly, so I disclosed that I have chronic fatigue syndrome, which is similar to Judy's illness. This seemed to build a bridge of common experience between us. I hoped that the disclosure would enhance our connection so that Judy could begin to trust me with her story.

A potential problem with therapist disclosure of an illness is that the client, concerned about the therapist's health, will be reticent about sharing her pain. She may come to believe that she is adding to the therapist's burden or that the therapist is too ill to bear the full impact of the client's story. Judy consistently expressed her concern about me, frequently inquiring about my health. I chose to answer these questions honestly, but without great detail. In order to maintain the focus on Judy and her needs, I reassured her that my needs were being met outside the relationship and that she did not need to take care of me.

HOME HEALTH CARE BENEFITS STOP

A month later, benefits, human resources, and corporate management at Lerner's employer joined forces with the managed care company to cut off Lerner's home health care. Reid-Cunningham and Lerner worked with Lerner's doctors to put in place a plan of action to ensure the continuity of Lerner's care.

> *LERNER*: In the weeks that followed my first meeting with Maureen, I began to thank my proverbial lucky stars that she had been referred. For the first time ever, I had felt totally helpless, alone, abandoned, and very scared in a city far away from home. My managed care plan was cutting me off at the knees (ironic given my accident), and my employer, to whom I had devoted virtually all my waking hours for years, traveling the world, working nights and weekends, delivering top-notch work and major business sales, was deserting me in my time of greatest need.
>
> But not Maureen. This stranger, this woman who walked into my bedroom as my guardian angel, didn't waste time. She got down to business. She listened to me. She heard my biggest concerns and she acted on them.
>
> My experience in life had contrasted sharply with the acceptance and responsiveness that I experienced with Maureen. In my family, I was never good enough, despite "A" grades and a record of stellar behavior. My teachers, while praising me, also learned to take my performance for granted. And then employers, seeing the level of production of which I was capable, demanded ever greater dedication and results, always expecting more and never leaving room for human frailty.
>
> As a perfectionist, I had developed a reputation for being difficult. Maureen quickly identified my strengths, reinforced my best qualities,

accepted my weaknesses, and let me know that, for better or worse, she was on my side. I felt heard.

In addition, although I wouldn't know how important this would become until months later, Maureen understood invisible, chronic illness. She shared this experience. So even before I identified consciously the effects my injury and benefits battles were having on my health, Maureen began to pinpoint symptoms and provide supportive tips on how to cope.

Just as important, Maureen was proactive to the extreme, a good fit with the overachiever in me (how she does that I will never know, given her own limitations due to chronic fatigue syndrome). For example, in the month between the first benefits skirmishes and full-out war, Maureen started discussions about a game plan for the inevitable home health care cutoff that was to come. When the ax finally fell, we were somewhat prepared.

The fateful news came on a Friday afternoon. With no warning, I got a call from the managed care plan (case manager and social worker) and my employer (benefits manager and human resources manager): a four-on-one attack. They called to announce that in a week, my 24-hour-a-day home care would be reduced to two hours a day and, a week later, to no care at all. Finding out that my surgeon was going on vacation that day, I asked for a reprieve until he returned. They refused. Their only concession: they would hold a conference call the following week with my primary care physician (standing in for the surgeon), my physical therapist, and Maureen to discuss my case.

No matter what I said, they argued. I finally explained that I was too upset to go on with the call and hung up. A minute later, two of them called back. I hung up again. Late that night, the two called again and, once more, I refused to talk. In my fragile state, they not only ignored my emotional distress, but called late at night to argue some more.

Maureen responded quickly once more. She helped to formulate a plan by which I would enlist my housekeeper, some home health aides and some agencies to provide continued home care, for which I would pay. Fortunately, I had the financial resources to do this. I would have the care necessary for my own medical well-being and safety. I could appeal the denial of benefits later.

The following week, Maureen joined my physical therapist and primary care physician on a conference call with the managed care plan and my employer's representatives. The call lasted nearly two hours. Two amazing warriors fought for me: Maureen and Cambridge, Massachusetts internist and Harvard professor Matthew Carmody, M.D. Even in this harried era of managed care, they took the time to argue patiently the medical and psychological rationale for ongoing home health care. They thought the managed care plan understood. They were wrong. These two spent the next year and a half by my side, expending innumerable hours writing letters, making phone calls, and coordinating with each other to ensure the preservation of my safety, my health, and my stand in the war for the benefits I deserved.

In the end, my home health care was cut off, and home health aides continued on a privately paid basis. Maureen and my physician never deserted me.

REID-CUNNINGHAM: The therapeutic connection was vital for Judy: it became her lifeline when everything else was spinning out of control. This put me, as the therapist, in a particularly powerful position. The balance of power in the therapeutic relationship is inevitably skewed in favor of the therapist who is being paid for her time and expertise. Addressing the power inequity became a part of the therapy (Hillyer, 1993; Jordan, 1991).

One of my goals in this therapy was for Judy to become empowered to care for herself, to feel that she was entitled to care, and to reach out to others for genuine connection and mutual relationships. She could articulate this goal, but she often believed it unattainable. Her recent experiences with disconnections and violations had left her feeling hurt and hopeless. In spite of this, she was able to connect with me and trust me when I reassured her that she would not always feel so isolated, vulnerable, and fearful.

I recognized that, by taking on this role, I was claiming a certain type of power over the relationship. It would have been easy to use this to distance myself from Judy's pain. Reassuring her that it would all turn out all right without acknowledging the very real problems she faced would have caused a disconnection in the relationship, perpetuating the pattern of Judy alone against the world. It became important to maintain a clear and realistic view of her difficult reality, while continuing to offer hope.

Prior to her injury, Judy had relied heavily upon her ability to produce superior work to establish and maintain her relationships. This was the case in childhood, when she received parental attention she needed in response to excelling in school and behavior, and in her adult life, when she devoted herself to professional achievement in order to attain validation and a sense of self worth. Because her relationships were based on what she could do, rather than on who she was, Judy's relational style proved painfully ineffective when she became unable to work.

This pattern of behavior represented what Miller and Stiver (1997) describe as the central relational paradox, in which an individual's strategies for connection with others actually result in disconnection. The therapeutic relationship provided opportunities for Judy to develop new strategies for developing meaningful, mutual relationships with others (Brown, 1986; Miller and Stiver, 1997).

THE RETURN TO WORK

Three and a half months after the accident, Lerner returned to work. Her surgeon was required to submit a "Physical Capabilities" form in advance, and he noted her limitations: no lifting, no bending, minimal walking, limited standing, and no more than three hours a day sitting and working. He recommended "telecommuting as much as possible" and special parking or transportation arrangements. Lerner's employer never discussed accommodating these limits.[5] In fact, she received increased pressure to perform and to be in the office full time.[6]

> *LERNER*: When I went back to work my own manager as well as our office manager didn't see me for three days. One was out of the office, the other out of sight.
>
> When we finally met, they said that in spite of a three and a half month absence, my performance goals would not be adjusted. "The goals are the goals." Moreover, if I didn't use up five weeks of vacation by year end, I would lose it. A classic no-win dilemma: take vacation or lose it while trying to meet virtually impossible performance goals in the last three months of the year. I opted to take vacation but felt my employer's betrayal to be complete.
>
> My new life was beginning to take shape. Never again would I sacrifice my own life and needs to meet an employer's expectations. I would protect myself first.
>
> In spite of my surgeon's recommendations, no accommodations were made to help me return to work. For example, I had a handicapped parking placard, but to get a space in the one block of handicapped parking beside our office tower, I had to arrive by 6:45 every morning. And as Boston winter approached, I found myself slugging through wind, rain, ice, and snow juggling a brief case, a cane, and an umbrella. By the time I reached my desk at seven each morning, I was already exhausted.
>
> My reputation for being a tough perfectionist escalated. Though I didn't know it yet, my fibromyalgia had begun to worsen after the accident as the stress of work took its toll. My memory and concentration worsened; my patience disappeared; my irritability grew. I heard that others found it difficult to deal with me.

The sinister part of fibromyalgia is that the worse cognitive and mood difficulties become, the harder it is for the patient to recognize them. So, I kept trying. And, I kept doing worse. I felt dejected, defeated, and alone.

Maureen, however, explained what was happening. She observed me and she heard about my treatment at work. She helped me to see that I needn't take all the responsibility. My employer was making life more (not less) difficult so soon after my accident.

Although I was now mobile, Maureen continued to come to my house for our therapy sessions, though I worried she would tell me to come to her office. By then, I had all I could do to get back and forth to work and survive each day. Any extra burden would put me over the edge.

REID-CUNNINGHAM: My personal experience with chronic illness continued to be an important part of our connection. Judy seemed to find it beneficial that I knew about chronic illness from both personal and professional perspectives. While the common threads of our experience were important, it was also necessary to recognize the uniqueness of each of our experiences and to understand that Judy must find her own ways to cope. I could offer advice based on what I knew, and she could decide whether or not that advice was a good fit for her.

I continued to see Judy at home for several reasons. It seemed important to meet her where she was, both clinically and concretely. Home visits provided an opportunity to care for and to nurture Judy. I hoped that, over time, Judy would begin to feel that she deserved such care and that she would improve her self-care skills. In addition, she was quite ill. Traveling to my office would have been a strain for her.

CHRONIC ILLNESS TAKES ITS TOLL

By January of 1997, the demands from Lerner's employer coupled with the "flare" of her fibromyalgia brought her to the brink of suicide. Reid-Cunningham and Carmody stepped in, pulling Lerner out on a short-term disability leave of absence from work. At home, Lerner began to write. Her passion, put aside long ago, would help sow the seeds of her future life.

LERNER: Pressures at work grew in January along with my weakness: unbearable fatigue, horrible muscle pain, "fog" in my head, uncontrollable mood swings, and more. I had to travel to Atlanta for a training course and barely held my head up for three days. Then, a client asked that I be taken off an assignment, the first time I had ever been fired by a client. Relationships with colleagues became more strained.

At the end of January, my manager held a closed-door session in which she told me, in essence, to shape up. She didn't believe my problems had any connection with my medical condition. Then she dumped a new project with a tight deadline in my lap.

I walked out of her office in a fog. I couldn't take any more. I packed my brief case and went home early. I called Maureen and told her I couldn't live this way anymore.

Maureen came quickly to my side. She conferred with my physician, who a month earlier had identified that the increasingly severe symptoms of fibromyalgia were doing damage and that without some respite from work, I would be in trouble. The two of them insisted I take a disability leave from work.

I called my manager and told her. She responded indignantly that I needed to complete my new assignment and ordered me to speak with the office head. My manager's punitive attitude felt like a knife in my side. I really wanted to die. Work had defined me. I had always been a success. Now no matter what I did, I seemed to fail.

Over the coming weeks, Maureen and my physician spent time providing reassurance. In frequent office visits, my physician focused not just on my body, but on my state of mind. The two of them taught me that the problems building up at work were not my fault. I had an illness, a real physical illness, affecting my behavior and my head. With their help, I began to make the transition from understanding fibromyalgia on an intellectual level to accepting it emotionally. With them to reinforce my strengths, I started down a path that would allow me to remain the smart, achievement-oriented woman I had always been, albeit in a different setting.

I found all my relationships altered. Fibromyalgia, an invisible illness, has little recognition and acceptance by the general public. Few understand it. Fewer know how difficult it is to live with. Friends and colleagues who had flocked to my door with flowers and sympathy after the accident stayed away. A psychologist I had seen years earlier labeled my illness "controversial." He had missed the implications of my physical symptoms: in the midst of severe depression, he told me to get a hobby. Invalidation overwhelmed me. It took Maureen, and her own experience with chronic illness, to help me see that others' denial of my condition was their problem, not mine.

At the same time, people I would never have expected rallied to my side. Some friendships strengthened and new ones formed. Faced with time on my hands and little energy, my mind raced. In my head, I began to relive a romantic drama I had imagined years earlier. I found myself thinking in sentences, then paragraphs. One morning, I went to my computer and began to write. A month later, I had a rough draft of a novel. I loved writing.

As a child, I had written poetry. In my teens, I lived my feelings on paper. But, I had put aside personal writing for the challenges of career. Now, I rediscovered my writing passion. It occurred to me that my battles with the benefits world had become a saga worth recording. I turned my notes into a journal, added tips on fighting managed care plans, and started a new book. Later, a top New York agent would accept me as a client.

As I completed drafts, I asked Maureen if she would like to read them. She eagerly said "yes." She became a fan, encouraging more writing and reacting both to my story and my craft. Maureen was hearing me as others never had before.

REID-CUNNINGHAM: Judy's return to work became a disaster for her, both emotionally and physically. She reported feeling suicidal, and her physician and I agreed that she needed time away from the damaging work situation. She greeted our joint recommendation that she apply for short-term disability with relief, although it was a difficult decision for her. She struggled against feelings that taking a disability leave represented failure at work, where she had always been competent and successful.

We talked a great deal about how she could regain the sense that she was a capable, powerful woman who could make choices about her life. Writing became her path back from her suicidal thoughts. The more she wrote, the stronger she became. I chose to read what Judy had written because I wanted to encourage her to use her genuine voice in any way that felt right for her and because it allowed additional access to her internal process. We incorporated discussions of her writing in therapy, providing another way to understand Judy's life experiences and their impact on her emotional and physical well-being.

DISABILITY BENEFITS DENIAL THREATENS SURVIVAL

After two and a half months on short-term disability, Lerner received notice that her disability benefits had been denied retroactively. Another war began. Not only would short-term disability benefits be denied, but long-term disability benefits as well. Lerner faced financial disaster.

LERNER: I received regular checks for short-term disability benefits. But then in April, a letter arrived saying my short-term disability claim had been denied back to January. I couldn't believe it. With no warning, my employer was cutting me off. The stated reason: my physician had failed to return phone calls about my status. This allegation proved false.

Two weeks of phone calls and angry letters from Maureen, my physician, my employer, the benefits administrator and me got short-term disability benefits reinstated. But I knew it was only a matter of time before another attempt would be made to cut me off.

My surgeon had scheduled a June surgery to remove the hardware from my broken legs. Given the benefits wars, I asked to advance surgery to May. It would be tough to deny disability benefits for surgery that would confine me for several weeks. Now benefits were driving health care decisions.

Surgery took place in May. Short-term disability benefits continued through June. At the end of June, five months into short-term disability, disability benefits were cut off permanently. I was not surprised. If I received six months of short-term disability payments, then my employer would be forced to consider my claim for long-term disability benefits which start in month six and could continue for the duration of disability. That could be an expensive proposition. In this managed care world, saving money is what it's all about.

I appealed. Maureen, my physician, my surgeon and others wrote strong appeal letters and provided substantial medical proof, but to no avail. In the end, I had to hire an attorney and eventually file suit.

The continuing benefits battles brought me down again and again. Terminating disability benefits would put me in serious financial jeopardy. I began to have visions of being a homeless person with a long string of shopping carts to hold my extensive business wardrobe.

Over and over, Maureen helped me to keep doom away from the door. She helped me see that my fears need not materialize. She urged me to work through options and create game plans for surviving adversity. In the end, those plans enabled me to move back home to Los Angeles.

REID-CUNNINGHAM: Judy's decision to move to Los Angeles demonstrated that she was ready to end her therapy with me and build a life that included not only her chronic illness, but mutual relationships and writing. She assumed a proactive, powerful stance and began to believe that she could handle anything else that life threw her way. She had learned to ask for help without feeling shame.

THE ADVOCATE IS BORN

As events unfolded, Lerner's activities and writing taught her more about the plight of others wrongfully denied their benefits. She realized her expertise could be used to fight for changes in laws and regulations.

> *LERNER*: After first my medical and then disability benefits were denied, I wondered what happens to the average person wrongfully denied benefits. After all, I was an expert in the field who knew the law, the regulations, the issues, the questions to ask, and the people with whom to talk. And I couldn't get through the system. I concluded that most Americans don't have a prayer. I wondered what I could do to change that.
>
> My book took shape. *Dead on Arrival: How to Survive HMOs, PPOs, and Benefit Woes* told my story from the date of the accident to one year later. Each section used my tale to illustrate what to do, with tips on how to survive and win against a health care and insurance system that has forgotten patients' needs.
>
> *Business and Health* magazine published my article, "The New Direction in Disability Management," in October 1998. It emphasized the human face of disability and the need to manage disability benefits with compassion. In April, 1999, *Business and Health* profiled my case in an article titled, "When the System Breaks Down."
>
> In 1998, I wrote to members of Congress about my personal experience, emphasizing that, as a former insider in the world of employee benefits, I had been unable to get the benefits due me. In the summer of 1998, I testified before a Congressional committee considering the "Patients' Bill of Rights." My testimony was shown on the NBC Nightly News. KCET's "Life and Times" and Fox 11 News did follow-up features. In every appearance, the message was this: the law must be changed to provide protection to those wrongly denied medical and disability benefits.[7]

POSTSCRIPT

Lerner now lives in a suburb of Los Angeles with her significant other. She still suffers the effects of fibromyalgia, having both good days and bad. She remains on Social Security disability benefits, managing her finances carefully.

> *LERNER*: For the first time in my life, I feel really good about myself. Throughout my long ordeal, I learned invaluable lessons about what

disability looks and feels like, about the struggles others face with physical incapacity and financial strain, about humanity and inhumanity, about the values and the people most important to me. Unable still to work, I miss the clients, but I don't miss the strife of office politics and corporate greed.

Through this experience, I have met incredible people. While pursuing my advocacy role, I connected with physicians, attorneys, and consumer experts with amazing drive and dedication; they have become my supporters and my friends. I have also formed relationships with people who would never have crossed my path had I remained on the corporate treadmill.

My purpose has changed. I live to live, not to work. The energy I have I devote to the people I love, to advocacy, and to writing in that order. That makes me content.

And I like myself. I have discovered both my strengths and my weaknesses, and I accept them both. These qualities make me a better person.

None of this would have been possible without Maureen. As a woman, a chronic illness sufferer, a dedicated therapist, and a warm and loving human being, she pointed the way out of some very dark caverns that seemed to have no exit. She lifted me up from the depths and showed me the light. I owe her my life.

NOTES

1. Fibromyalgia falls into the classification of chronic, invisible illnesses for which as yet there is no known cause and no found cure. Like chronic fatigue syndrome, lupus, multiple sclerosis, and chronic lyme disease, fibromyalgia has symptoms that can include extreme fatigue, muscle pain, cognitive difficulties, and irritable bowel syndrome. The diagnosis of fibromyalgia involves the identification through palpitation of "tender points"–18 locations that produce pain on touch and that generally are raised, swollen, or knotted tissue; to be diagnosed officially with fibromyalgia, a patient must have 11 of the 18 tender points, with at least one in each of the four body quadrants (left, right, upper, and lower).

2. Her legal case has now been resolved out of court.

3. I had coverage in a "PPO" (preferred provider organization). Translation: I could go to any doctor or hospital, but my benefits would be higher using those that were part of the plan. And lest you think I had full freedom of choice, remember that virtually all medical plans today are managed. That is, the plan has the right to determine whether a medical service is "medically necessary" or whether it is covered by the plan; if the answer is "no," the plan won't pay. For most Americans, who can't afford to pay for care on their own, denied benefits mean denied care.

4. Miller and Stiver (1997) describe " . . . connections–the experience of mutual engagement and empathy."

5. Under the Americans with Disabilities Act, accommodations must be made for employees with injuries and illnesses (including mental and psychological impairments) that meet specific criteria unless accommodation would pose significant financial jeopardy.

6. As a consultant, Lerner normally spent more than half her time out of the office traveling and working at client locations. And like many of her colleagues, she often worked at home when she needed quiet in order to concentrate. Thus, her request to work at home some days following the accident actually fit into the "normal" scheme of things.

7. Federal law–ERISA (the Employee Retirement Income Security Act of 1974) governs all employer-provided benefits. Under ERISA, when a benefit is denied, you can sue only for the amount of benefits denied no matter how egregious the violation of law or how dire the consequences. So if medical benefits denied result in major health damage or even death, no compensatory or punitive damages are allowed. Without the threat of damage awards, managed care plans and their employer sponsors have no incentive to comply.

AUTHOR NOTES

Judy R. Lerner, born and raised in Los Angeles, California, spent nearly 20 years as a consultant in human resources communication, helping major companies communicate key corporate issues and also their benefit programs. She had been a Principal at some of the top firms in her business, serving major corporations and health care organizations. Ironically, she had specialized in helping companies and health care organizations install managed care plans. She moved to the Boston area for career reasons, far from family and lifetime friends, a year before her accident.

Maureen Reid-Cunningham, LICSW, BCD, is a clinical social worker with over 25 years' experience in the human services field. She currently has a private practice in Cambridge, Massachusetts, and has worked with many women who live with chronic illness. Maureen belongs to the Study Group on Women and Chronic Illness, which focuses on the impact of illness on women's lives and strategies women use to find meaning in an altered existence. She developed a chronic illness, Chronic Fatigue Syndrome, over twelve years ago.

REFERENCES

Brown, L. S. (1986). From alienation to connection: Feminist therapy with post-traumatic stress disorder. *Women & Therapy, (5)1,* 13-26.

Gemignani, J. (1999). When the system breaks down. *Business and Health, (17)4,* 21-25.

Hillyer, B. (1993). *Feminism and disability.* Norman, OK: University of Oklahoma Press.

Jordan, J. (1981). The movement of mutuality and power. *Work in Progress No. 53.* Wellesley, MA: Stone Center Working Papers Series.

Lerner, J. R. (1997). *Dead on arrival: How to survive HMOs, PPOs and benefit woes.* Unpublished manuscript.

Lerner, J. R. (1998). The new direction in disability management. *Business and Health, (16)10,* 21-25.

Miller, J. B. and Stiver, I. P. (1997). *The healing connection: How women form relationships in therapy and in life.* Boston: Beacon Press.

Reid-Cunningham, M., Snyder-Grant, D., Stein, K., Tyson, E., and Halen, B. (1999). Women with chronic illness: Overcoming disconnection. *Work in Progress No. 80.* Wellesley, MA: Stone Center Working Paper Series.

Social Construction of Illness:
Addressing the Impact of Cancer
on Women in Therapy

Suni Petersen
Lois A. Benishek

SUMMARY. There is no question that a diagnosis of cancer has a significant impact on anyone, however, certain aspects of American culture and particularly the medical culture exacerbate the impact. This article supports the notion that a woman's experience of cancer is, at least in part, socially constructed, political in nature, and therefore, uniquely disempowering to women. Those cultural forces affecting women with cancer include the stigma, the socially-embedded self-definitions, and the practices that dominate the medical-industrial complex. This article demonstrates how the use of social constructivist therapy can assist women in disengaging from these cultural forces while engaging in new ways of thinking and behaving that, in empirical studies, have resulted in decreased progression of disease, longer survival rates, and more effective coping with cancer. *[Article copies available for a fee from The Haworth Document Delivery Service: 1-800-342-9678. E-mail address: <getinfo@haworthpressinc.com> Website: <http://www.Haworth Press.com>* © *2001 by The Haworth Press, Inc. All rights reserved.]*

KEYWORDS. Cancer, empowerment, social constructivism, therapy and illness

---

Suni Petersen and Lois A. Benishek are Assistant Professors in the Department of Psychological Studies in Education, Counseling Psychology Program at Temple University. All correspondence regarding this article should be directed to Suni Petersen, 270 A Weiss Hall (265-63), Counseling Psychology Program, Temple University, Philadelphia, PA 19122 (E-mail: petersen@astro.temple.edu).

[Haworth co-indexing entry note]: "Social Construction of Illness: Addressing the Impact of Cancer on Women in Therapy." Petersen, Suni, and Lois A. Benishek. Co-published simultaneously in *Women & Therapy* (The Haworth Press, Inc.) Vol. 23, No. 1, 2001, pp. 75-100; and: *Minding the Body: Psychotherapy in Cases of Chronic and Life-Threatening Illness* (ed: Ellyn Kaschak) The Haworth Press, Inc., 2001, pp. 75-100. Single or multiple copies of this article are available for a fee from The Haworth Document Delivery Service [1-800-342-9678, 9:00 a.m. - 5:00 p.m. (EST). E-mail address: getinfo@haworthpressinc.com].

In reaction to the dehumanizing, stigmatizing, and degrading politicized metaphors that ascribe cultural meaning to illness, cancer being one, Susan Sontag and others have made a plea to abolish all cultural metaphors regarding illness (Lupton, 1995; Sontag, 1989). Talcott Parsons (1972), also recognizing the politics of illness, suggested that medicine is a form of sanctioned deviancy, a rebellion against that which is oppressive, and as such, not metaphoric but actualized resistance. We contend that the cultural metaphor for illness is political and as inescapable as doing therapy without consideration for the fact that our theories and words are laden with values. However, we believe it is just that—a metaphor. Furthermore, since metaphors are constructions of people, they can and should be changed in the therapeutic process with women who have been diagnosed with cancer.

People live by metaphors. Metaphors are ways of extracting the essence of many interacting stimuli and organizing them in a coherent, meaningful way. Metaphors are provided for us, often as children, as we are socialized into the culture in which we live. They are based on unquestioned assumptions, are usually accepted as "truths," and, therefore, often go unquestioned. Existing cultural metaphors frame our interpretation of experience. These unquestioned "truths" direct attention to certain aspects of the experience while excluding other aspects of the experience. This, in turn, results in selective perceptions that reflect the culture.

These "truths" remain unexamined because they are never spoken. While a person might be somewhat aware of the cultural metaphor, the intermediating, ensuing assumptions are relegated to obscurity. Although unlanguaged experience remains unexamined, it does not mean the person is untouched by the gestalt of that experience. Conceptualization is grounded in spatial experience, physical sensation and a vast background of cultural presuppositions (Maturana & Varella, 1987). However, there is a distinction between conception and experience (Lakoff & Johnson, 1980).

Experience is a direct interaction with the physical environment and bodily sensation. Experience can occur without language. Take, for example, date rape, an experience that offers enough ambiguity in the definition that it is not immediately represented in language. The experience is real and is attributed with great significance. Yet it remains without words or definition often until hours, days, or months later. It is not that the experience does not hold significance or that the victim is unaware of the significance prior to the labeling. Decisions are made relative to that experience even before the label occurs. For instance, the rape victim may avoid men or may be too afraid to leave her home. The experience, therefore, has great meaning in the person's life without the linguistic construction of the definition of "date rape." People's constructions of illness, specifically cancer, occur in the same way.

Cancer is an insidious disease. Tumors begin to grow unbeknownst to the person. Early signs of cancer are easily excused because they are not inter-preted as symptoms. Pain, extreme fatigue, swelling, discoloration, charac-teristics usually associated with symptoms, are not present and thereby allow for no prediagnosis preparation for the "experience" of cancer. The experi-ence of cancer is the physical sensation; the conception of cancer is the labeling of an experience and the meaning attributed based on cultural pre-suppositions. A woman recently diagnosed with cancer is often given the label of cancer before having the associated physical experiences. The label and the socially-constructed meaning of cancer precedes her actual physical, spatial, and social experience. Furthermore, the label is imposed on her by the medical system and the meaning is initially imposed upon her by the prevail-ing cultural expectations for the disease. Therefore, the internal experience is one of unwanted intrusion on her life by the cancer and often experienced as an intrusion from both the diagnosing system and cultural images.

THE CULTURALLY-CONSTRUCTED MEDICAL SYSTEM

Like other institutions, the medical system operates within a cultural meta-phor. Both the medical system and the illness, itself, are wrapped in a bundle of unassailable assumptions that stem from this guiding metaphor. The guid-ing metaphors are reflected in both the language and the actions surrounding healing in Western society.

The prevailing metaphor of Western medicine is "medicine is science" (Acterberg, 1990). This metaphor serves several functions. First, the medical system is one of the institutional fruits of capitalism and, as such, is guided by the business of medicine. Hospitals, medical insurers, pharmaceutical com-panies, and cost-watchdog businesses are major industries whose interests center around their own profits. The "medicine is science" metaphor hides the fact that medicine is business. Economic watch-dogging denies some patients certain treatments as medical institutions answer to stock holders. The emergence of resource-based relative value scales restrict practice to standard formulas assigned by an external source. Alliances are constructed and then de-constructed within a nexus of practice arrangements between insurers, hospitals, and businesses. The regulatory component of medicine has shifted from government domination to corporate domination, diminish-ing public control (Hafferty & Light, 1995). In our capitalistic society, the "medicine is science" metaphor serves to uphold exclusionary practices, retain a power elite, and control resources. High rates of infant mortality, absence of a cure for two leading diseases (i.e., heart disease and cancer), failing to decrease the spread of infectious disease, such as AIDS, and virtually ignor-ing ailments afflicting minorities are examples of this.

"Medicine as science" has also led to the split between mind and body and the growth of allopathic medicine. This split is a gendered concept. As men took over the science of healing the body, a single monolithic system was built that forbade by law all other forms of healing practices and subjected women to working in submissive, conforming roles vis-a-vis the male dominated profession. Even today with women entering the medical field in increasingly higher numbers and positions (Stacey, 1994), as they do, the feminization of certain practice areas is followed by a decrease in income and value associated with that specialty (Turner, 1995). Because American medical training claims to be scientific in nature, the "Medicine as science" metaphor supports the following assumptions: (1) American medicine is the best in the world; (2) the physician is and should be objective and because of the objectivity knows what is best for the patient; and (3) the use of invasive medical procedures and expensive technology should not be questioned.

"Medicine as science" is based on reductionistic methods that promote another metaphor for treating the body, i.e., "body as a machine." This metaphor suggests that the body can be separated into its parts and that doing so will allow the broken parts to be fixed. The study of treating people became the study of diseased parts rather than understanding and facilitating the body's natural healing abilities. Disease is seen as a problem to be tackled from outside, thus justifying an active, sometimes aggressive approach. Such a metaphor naturally led to the development of harsh chemicals that target a particular locale so that its "active ingredients" could affect change. This was done by minimizing the side effects of those ingredients on other areas of the body. Evidence supporting other treatments, such as natural botanics, are ignored because they are unscientific, unprofitable, and often positively affect more than just the problem under treatment. This zero-sum environment is the context under which women are being treated in our current medical system.

Within any culture, the patient is also provided with a metaphor for illness. In Western medicine, the metaphor is revealed in language such as, "battling the disease," "victim of disease," and "attacked by a virus." The metaphor is "illness is a malevolent enemy" (Acterberg, 1990) and as such, can only be fought with an attack. From the patient's position, she is told she has a disease (e.g., cancer), and the "science of medicine" will provide the chemical warfare to attack the disease. In the midst of the raging war between the chemotherapy injected in her veins and the insidious onslaught of cancer, the patient is expected to remain relatively calm and passively obedient while "fighting her disease." Exactly what does that mean? How is that possible? And where does the "science of medicine" and the "disease as enemy" leave women, when they have already been subjected to the cultural presuppositions that women are not scientific and cannot/should not fight?

Western constructions disempower women by perpetuating negative images of illness, in general, and cancer, in particular. These images are associated with the "wretchedness" of cancer-related deaths, cancer's mutilating nature, its ability to "attack without warning," and its unpredictability regarding progression and treatment outcomes (Peters-Golden, 1982). Receiving a diagnosis of cancer is more stigmatizing than receiving a diagnosis of many other chronic illnesses (Allbrecht, Walker, & Levy, 1982; Patterson, 1987; Stahly, 1988).

Stigma is defined as a "negative evaluation linked to characteristics of a person, which places the person outside some socially accepted standard for human attributes or performance" (Bloom & Kessler, 1994, p. 119). It stems from the Greek practice of branding slaves who unsuccessfully attempted to escape from their masters with the letter, F, for fugitive [Funk, 1950, as cited in Weiner, Perry, & Magnusson (1988)]. The word for such a mark was stigma. This "mark" identifies the individual as being "deviant, flawed . . . spoiled or generally undesirable" (Jones, Farina, Hastort, Markus, Miller, & Scott, 1984, p. 6). It is no wonder that the term cancer is "often the metaphor chosen for any social state or condition that slowly but inexorably destroys or erodes . . . such . . . as 'the cancer of our society' . . . conveys its sinister meaning and contributes to the stigmatization of the person who has cancer" (Holland, 1991, p. 4).

Historically, a diagnosis of cancer was synonymous with receiving a death sentence. Contagion fears were rampant (Apfel, Love, & Kalinowski, 1994; Batt, 1994; Bloom & Kessler, 1994), and people did not talk openly about the topic. "Cancer was . . . a condition to which a superstitious dread adhered, as well as a rational and understandable fear–to talk about it was to invoke it, to speak briefly or in a lowered voice was to leave it sleeping" (Blaxter, 1983, p. 41 as cited in Featherstone, 1996). The 1960s brought a slightly more hopeful perspective about cancer which, in large part, was due to developments in cancer treatments and the resulting potential for cure (Holland, 1992). In the decade of the 1970s, a California survey described by Dagrosa (1980) indicated that cancer was more feared than either violent crimes or atomic war. Information dissemination and the resulting heightened awareness about cancer served to decrease the stigma and fear associated with cancer at about this time (Sontag, 1989). The impact of the feminist movement was witnessed in the 1980s with increased attention being paid to the impact of language on women's perception of chronic illness and cancer (Lorde, 1980; Sontag, 1989). Most recently, greater emphasis is being placed on strengths, coping, and survivorship of women with cancer (Meyerowitz, Chaiken, & Clark, 1988; Nezu, Nezu, Friedman, Faddis, & Houts, 1999).

Despite positive changes, substantial evidence indicates that negative attitudes and stigma associated with receiving a diagnosis of cancer prevail. Misinformation and stigma appear to remain problematic among certain subgroups of individuals (Bloom, Grazier, Hodge, & Hayes, 1991). For example, 63% of one sample of African American women associated a diagnosis of cancer with a death sentence and believed that cancer was contagious (as cited in Bloom & Kessler, 1994). The medical community also appears to continue to have stigmatized constructions of cancer given that medical professionals ascribe more negative images to cancer than do their patients (Heuser, 1991).

There is some indication that the feminist movement is responsible for the lessening of cancer-related stigma and changes in the negative constructions of cancer that have occurred over time. It is noteworthy that the stigma appears to be decreasing for the more "feminine" types of cancer (e.g., breast cancer) in which women have focused considerable effort and provided education about cancer prevention and treatment. Feminists are outspoken about the emotional damage that results from adhering to male constructions of health and femininity (Bricker-Jenkins, 1994; Wilkinson & Kitzinger, 1994). The stigma is being challenged by qualitative research efforts and an increase in biographical accounts written by and about women with cancer (e.g., Bricker-Jenkins, 1994; Datan, 1989; Keith, 1991; Lorde, 1980). Advocacy efforts are giving voice to these women and providing them with opportunities to become more aware not only of the ways in which culture imposes its constructions of cancer upon them, but also in the ways in which they, themselves, can reconstruct those images to be personally meaningful and empowering.

WHY ARE THE CULTURAL IMAGES OF CANCER PARTICULARLY DISEMPOWERING FOR WOMEN?

Broad cultural images of women are centered around several themes: (1) women as sexual partners, (2) women as caretakers and nurturers of others, and (3) women as source of reproduction. It is not by accident that the female archetype is also the feminine stereotype of a patriarchal society. These images are thrust on women. Those who do not comply are considered less female; those who comply are elevated as models (MacKinnon, 1989). The meaning behind these images equate the feminine with a certain innate vulnerability which allows easy sexual access, passivity and disabled resistance, reinforced by trained physical weakness and softness (MacKinnon, 1989). "The overall objective of female conditioning is to make women perceive themselves and their lives through male eyes and so to secure the unquestioning acceptance of a male-defined and male-derived existence" (Brownmiller, 1975, p. 4).

Women's marginalized status in the world is exacerbated when they receive a diagnosis of cancer. Societal constructions of cancer center around the somewhat overlapping ideologies of the "just world" (Bloom & Kessler, 1994; Peters-Golden, 1982), "blaming the victim" (Sontag, 1989; Wilkinson & Kitzinger, 1994), and the "enlightenment" philosophies (Brickman, Rabinowitz, Karuza, Coates, Coh, & Kidder, 1982). These perspectives suggest that women, either consciously or subconsciously, are responsible for the development of their cancer. In essence, these ideologies place cancer within a "moral context" (i.e., cancer is the consequence of wrongful behaviors; Wilkinson & Kitzinger, 1994). Lupton's review of the popular media's construction of breast cancer provides a clear example of how women are portrayed as contributing to their diagnosis of breast cancer. These media reports suggested that women's entry into the employment world and the resulting delay in child bearing was linked to breast cancer. Although there is evidence to support the association between breast cancer and delaying childbirth (King, 1993), the implicit message to women was that there were dire consequences associated with shifting away from more traditional female roles.

Cultural images shape the numerous life roles and scripts that constitute women's identity. These roles and scripts are threatened when cancer is diagnosed. In essence, a diagnosis of cancer represents a "secondary victimization" (Brickman et al., 1982), which shifts women from their existing precarious sociocultural position to one of even greater vulnerability and disempowerment.

Women's roles as nurturer and caregiver are threatened. Surgery and adjuvant therapies result in nausea, fatigue, and limited physical mobility, which in turn, lead to role reversals. Women are faced with either temporarily or permanently relinquishing their caregiving activities and they struggle with allowing themselves to be cared for by others (Keller, Henrich, Sellschopp, & Beutel, 1996; Siegel, 1990; Thompson & Fits, 1992).

Women's sense of self as a sexual being is also impacted by the diagnosis. The diagnosis and treatment of cancer often results in decreased libido and sexual functioning (Anderson & Jochimsen, 1985; Ganz, 1998; Kaplan, 1992; Smith & Reilly, 1994). Spouses and life partners may also have difficulty adjusting to the diagnosis of cancer, as indicated by some partners' difficulty with sexual intimacy (Anderson, Anderson, & deProsse, 1989a; 1989b). Furthermore, cancer often results in physical changes to the woman's body. The surgical removal of a breast or breast tissue, a uterus, the loss of hair, changes in bone structure, as well as treatment-induced changes in skin texture and color all result in women having to reconstruct or reconfigure (sometimes literally) their sense of self. They may feel less sexual or desirable to their partner given these physical alterations. Their bodies–either internally or externally–no longer represent the same "self" that they (and others) have intimately interacted with during the course of their lifetime.

Related to women's sense of self as a sexual being, women's sense of self as a bearer of life is often temporarily or permanently altered. This occurs either as a direct consequence of the cancer (i.e., uterine cancer that results in a hysterectomy) or as an indirect consequence of the cancer (i.e., chemothera-py or oophorectomy which results in premature menopause). Certain types of cancer and/or its treatment leave women with no choice other than to sacri-fice their option to bear children.

Historically, women's expression of affect has been viewed in a negative light (i.e., the overly emotional woman; e.g., Cook, 1944). One would think that having strong emotional reactions to receiving a diagnosis of cancer would be perceived as "normal" in our society (Noyes & Kathol, 1986; Stefanek, Shaw, DeGeorge, & Tsottles, 1989). However, women are stigma-tized, penalized, and further disempowered when they respond with strong affect to their cancer diagnosis. "Appropriate" emotional reactions and our conceptions of mental health are also socially constructed by people in power (Conrad, 1980; Parker, Georgaca, Harper, McLaughlin & Stowell-Smith, 1995).

This disempowerment associated with women's expression of emotions happens in several ways. First, medical professionals often feel uncomfort-able with women's emotionality and either ignore their feelings (Lerman, Daly, Walsh, Resch et al., 1993) or attempt to contain them through the use of prescription medications (McBride, 1987). Second, family members are often uncomfortable with the woman's emotionality and either retreat from feelings (i.e., don't talk about the cancer; Sabo, Brown, & Smith, 1986) or minimize their relevance in the woman's life (Lichtman, Taylor, & Wood, 1988). Finally, some emotions (e.g., sadness, fear) are perceived as more acceptable than others (e.g., anger). Unfortunately, the more empowering affective reactions are viewed as less acceptable in our culture (Burtle, 1985). This is unfortunate given that the ability to express anger as a means of coping has been associated with less of a likelihood of developing cancer (Cooper & Faragher, 1993) and with greater longevity after receiving a diagnosis of cancer (Spiegel, Kraemer, Bloom, & Gottheil, 1989).

Paid employment has become an instrumental aspect of women's identi-ties as they have moved into the working world in record numbers. In com-parison to the 1930s when approximately 30% of the U.S. workforce con-sisted of women (Russo & Denmark, 1984), today almost 80% of women report working outside of the home (Betz, 1993).

Unfortunately, cancer treatment and the recovery process either temporari-ly or permanently impede women's ability to maintain their paid employment positions. Despite the passing of the Americans with Disabilities Act of 1990, employment discrimination still occurs, with women either being demoted, released from their jobs, or simply treated differently once co-workers and employers learn about their diagnosis (McCharen & Earp, 1981). Furthermore, work responsibilities can no longer be fulfilled if the cancer progresses. This results in women having to relinquish work roles that have led to a sense of personal fulfillment and financial independence.

In summary, the role changes that result from receiving a diagnosis of cancer can serve to further disempower women. Women's culturally-imposed roles coupled with a diagnosis of cancer result in women (and the world) viewing themselves as less than whole and as not able to fulfill their own personal and professional needs. As a result, they are less able to involve themselves in roles that they find meaningful and fulfilling. The nurturer becomes the nurtured, the sexual being becomes neutered, the bearer of life becomes sterile, the emotional woman becomes the hysterical woman, and the generative woman becomes stagnant. By examining the politics of these practices, the demeaning, dehumanizing, and stigmatizing metaphors and assumptions can be replaced by new, idiosyncratic, and empowering metaphors.

ILLNESS AS A SOCIALLY CONSTRUCTED PHENOMENON

Although the medical model pervades our health care system, women have increasingly embraced alternative perspectives to the bio-medical model both as consumers and practitioners (Achterberg, 1990). A growing body of empirical studies have documented that factors such as psychological adjustment (Kreitler, Kreitler, Chaitchik, Shaked, & Shaked, 1997), attitude (Pettingale, Morris, Greer, & Haybrittle, 1985), and active coping predict slower disease progression and survival with greater accuracy than medical criteria such as the stage of cancer (Derogatis, Abeloff, & Melisaratos, 1979; Epping-Jordan, Compas, & Howell, 1994; Jensen, 1987; Temoshek, 1985). Self-perceived pain was related more to depression (Banks & Kerns, 1996; Turk, Rudy, & Salovey, 1986) and cognitive distortion (Geisser, Robinson, Keefe, & Weiner, 1994; Smith, Christensen, Peck, & Ward, 1994) than physical evidence would lead one to expect. Those patients who used a biological explanation for their illness exhibited higher levels of impairment and poorer outcomes (Butler, Chalder, Ron, & Wessely, 1991; Ray, Jefferies, & Weir, 1995) than those who used idiosyncratic attributions. Studies on immune system functioning provide an even stronger link between psychological factors and physical determinants of illness (Dobbin, Harth, McCain et al., 1991; Esterling, Kiecolt-Glasser, Bodnar, & Glaser, 1994; Fawzy, Kemeny, Fawzy et al., 1990). Factors such as coping styles, attributions of causality, and active participation in important relationships have been associated with increases in natural killer cells. The results of these studies support a mind-body metaphor of disease (i.e., a psychological-biological model). However, the mind-body metaphor still retains the bias of an individualistic paradigm.

Great admiration is generated in our culture for the patient who "just goes on," "picks herself up," or "displays a strong attitude."

Investigations conducted on the relationship between social support and illness are beginning to challenge the strictly individual paradigm. However, biased by the individual paradigm, even these studies have tended to define social support as the functional and structural support of the patient; they are still embedded within the prevailing individual metaphor. Most studies on social support were conducted on men using the presence of a marital partner as a measure of social support. This method of assessing social support is predictive of recovery and survival in men but not in women (Brackett & Powell, 1988; Case, Moss, & Case et al., 1992; Ruberman, Weinblatt, & Goldberg et al., 1984). Most studies conducted on women found that being married is not predictive of ill health or recovery. Furthermore, several well-conducted studies demonstrated that marriage is actually a predictor of ill health in women (Cassileth, Lusk, & Miller et al., 1985; Waxler-Morrison, Hislop, & Mears, 1991).

Individualistic paradigms assess social support assuming that the process is linear and unidirectional. When measures of support are more inclusive and more reciprocal, positioning the patient within a social system, studies found reciprocity and full participation in relationships to be the critical feature in affecting health outcomes (Dimond, 1985; Power, 1979; Radley & Green, 1986; Stetz, Lewis, & Primono, 1988; Waltz, 1986; Worden, 1988).

The reciprocal nature of interactions with the environment operates to influence health outcomes through a social-cognitive process. The perception of seriousness and attribution of the illness to external causes were associated with more problems with physical functioning (Hiejmans & deRitter, 1998). People who engage in a reappraisal process over the course of an illness cope more effectively (Leventhal, Easterling, Coons, Luchterland, & Love, 1986), and experience less progression of disease and improved health outcomes (Epping-Jordan et al., 1994; Hiejmans & deRitter, 1998; Hilton, 1989). Key to the reappraisal process is the existence of a referent group of people with whom a patient identifies (Rodin, 1978). For men, the family frequently operates as the referent with whom to conduct this socially-engendered re-appraisal process. For women, marriage has frequently not served this purpose. Intimate relationships within which the re-appraisal can be conducted are outside their primary relationship (Antonucci, 1985; Goodwin, Hunt, & Samet, 1991; Rose, 1990; Waxler-Morrison et al., 1991) or within support groups, both of which have been found to influence not only the impact of the illness but also recovery (Bloom & Spiegel, 1984; Fawzy et al., 1993; Levy, Herberman, Sanzo, Lee, & Kirkwood, 1990).

Diagnosis and treatment are defined by a health care system reflecting the prevailing cultural metaphors, "illness is an individual problem that may be helped by medical science." Results of the aforementioned studies demonstrate that the direction of the individual's illness is affected, however, by her own psychology, the social situation in which she finds herself, and the physical nature of the illness. The results of these studies change the emphasis to a *socio-political*-psycho-bio model. The shift in emphasis makes clear the socio-political nature of labeling the disease and the treatment, rightly positioning the source of the labels outside the individual. Using a constructivist perspective invites the agenda of the labeler to be carefully scrutinized rather than blindly accepting the label. The constructivist view also establishes a new metaphor creating a necessary shift in the definition of illness (i.e., "illness as indicator of change"; "illness as a wake up call to reexamine one's environment.")

The constructivist perspective collapses the boundaries between mind, body, and culture, seeking multiple causes and, therefore, multiple sources of recovery as it defies conceptual neutrality on the part of any individual. The constructivist view means that (1) illness is context-bound, influenced by an individual's biology, an individual's psychology, and the social environment; (2) attributions of causality are based in theories and, as such, value-laden; (3) there is no absolute truth about an illness; and (4) the person(s) treating an illness and the person with the illness are inextricably bound through an interactive, self-influencing process. This process ultimately plays a significant role in the experience and progression of the illness and in some cases even survival. Illness, what the patient is doing about it, and how the illness is experienced is a product of the patient's constructions and these constructions have been derived from the socio-cultural context.

The patient's system of constructs (i.e., how she defines her illness, attributes causality, and attaches meaning to treatment) are superimposed on the "real world" of medicine. This "real world" of medicine is only indirectly reflected in the reality of healthcare workers. They, too, have a socially constructed reality that is thought to be superior to that of the patient because it is "scientifically based" and held in esteem by the dominant culture. This process of the professionals' construals being upheld as superior to lay people's construals is itself a social construction. From this point of view, "objective" is simply another subjective construal that is cloaked in the garb of an unattainable epistemic perfection. Patients whose own construals conflict with the "more objective" construal of the health care workers must either modify their construals in lock-step or face being labeled "noncompliant."

People accept this intellectual hegemony because it provides them with some degree of relief from the terror of feeling out of control of their bodies. When the cost of managing one's terror by giving up one's own construals is too high, the only option available is to repudiate the medical industrial complex's construals. Legitimacy is seldom granted to the experience of the patient when it conflicts with the metaphor of the medical system.

The medical system is composed of a tri-cultural terrain, the construals of the patient, those of the physician, and those of the institution in which treatment is delivered. "All belief systems are culture-bound because they are based on cultural factors and the meaning that individuals ascribe to their factors" (Bauwens & Anderson, 1993, p. 93). Being ill carries with it costs and benefits reflective of these cultural meanings. The costs and benefits are prescribed by the dominant culture's metaphor. There is an inherent inequity between men's and women's roles and positions; women are poorer and receive little support in their roles (Rodin & Ichovics, 1990; Scharf & Toole, 1992). Women typically juggle multiple roles within and outside their families (Scar, Phillips, & McCartney, 1989; Worell & Remer, 1992). In an effort to preserve their self-esteem, taking care of others precludes taking care of themselves, particularly when energy stores are low (Morrison, 1992). This is especially true in working class women (Cornwell, 1984). A woman simultaneously tries to be a "good patient" according to the medical system which means compliant with medical regimens, uncomplaining, responsive, and expending energy on self-care.

Attending physicians may be unaware of these inequities and aware of other inequities, such as the differences in coverage for women's conditions in comparison to men's conditions. In such instances, the physician is faced with challenging the medical system, their own institution, or third party payors. For instance, many insurers will reimburse for Viagra but not for birth control pills. Insurers do not pay for prophylactic mastectomies when the cost is $888 per quality-adjusted life year (compared to $27,300/quality-adjusted life year if she has metasticized breast cancer requiring a bone marrow transplant) (Grann, Panageas, Antman, & Neugut, 1998). However, bone marrow transplants are still considered experimental by third-party payors and women are seldom reimbursed for this treatment (King, 1993). Women, in particular, are caught in the web of these interacting cultural forces, increasing their sense of victimization.

How can we empower women by assisting them in reconstructing the meanings they attribute to receiving a diagnosis of cancer? Suzanne Pharr defines empowerment as "the ability to speak our own truths in our own voice and participate in decisions that affect our lives" (Pharr, 1988, p. 1 as cited in Bricker-Jenkins, 1994).

To the credit of the medical establishment, positive shifts have taken place in the recent past. These include policy changes regarding the disclosure of medical information that includes diagnostic information, prognosis, and treatment options (Pasacreta, McCorkle, & Margolis, 1991). For instance, approximately 90% of physicians did not inform their patients about their diagnosis of cancer in the 1950s (Oken, 1961) in comparison to 95% of physicians who did by the 1970s (Novack, Plumer, & Smith, 1979). Furthermore, women are more likely to be included in the decision-making process today than they were in the past (Gillespie, 1995; Holland, 1992).

Despite these positive changes, women continue to struggle to assess the impact of the illness on their lives and reconstruct it in a way that leads to their making a positive adjustment to their diagnosis. Recent studies indicate that patients desire more involvement in decision-making (Degner, Kristjanson, Bowman et al., 1997; Lerman, Biesecker, Benkendorf et al., 1997). Although women are taking a more active role than men in the decision-making process (Petersen, Heesacker, Schwartz, & Marsh, 2000), they are not necessarily communicating their needs to their attending physician, for instance, regarding seeking alternative medical regimens (Adler & Fosket, 1999; Begbie, Kerestes, & Bell, 1996).

SOCIAL CONSTRUCTIVIST APPROACH TO THERAPY WITH WOMEN FACED WITH A SERIOUS ILLNESS

Social constructivism is one theoretical strategy that can be used to promote greater empowerment in women who have been diagnosed with cancer. It is important to note that a constructivist approach recognizes the creative potential of adversity to result in positive life-changes. Therapists may believe that this is not the time for life changes. *We* propose that it is exactly the ideal time for significant life changes. This philosophy has been articulated by our clients with cancer who make statements such as, "Cancer was the best and worst thing that ever happened to me." This statement suggests that cancer provided an opportunity to identify unhealthy patterns in their lives and to summon the courage to change them. Support and coping are not enough to facilitate these changes, because only those coping strategies that fit within the woman's constructs are likely to be used and even those strategies may not generalize once the formal therapeutic experience is completed.

A construct is an image (visual or idea) that encompasses the entirety of an event. In addition to the constructs of the medical system, a patient also has constructs for the role of an ill person, how others are supposed to treat a person with illness, how much control over the illness a person has, and what behavior to engage in while undergoing treatment. Constructs concerning illness are often formulated without critical evaluation through vicarious experience (Berger & Luckman, 1966). A person's constructs determine both their interpretation of experience (Langer, Chanowicz, Palmerind, Jacobs, & Thayer, 1990) and behavior. It is, therefore, imperative to elicit and explore a woman's images of illness.

However, it is not only her images of illness, but also her images of herself, that influence how she copes with cancer. Parry and Doan (1994) suggest that subscribing to "a grand narrative" provided by the dominant culture allows for only one "self." To the degree that a woman accepts the dominant culture's view of who she is (this singular, stereotyped self), her options for coping with a life-threatening illness will be diminished. Efforts for coping and recovery must be restrained within the boundaries of whichever image of woman she has previously accepted. Additionally, adopting the cultural image as her own single identity dichotomizes behavior and cognitions into feminine/not feminine, me/not me, which also allows for a very limited range of behavior. This limited repetoire of behaviors will remain in place until she struggles with and becomes aware of her own enculturated illness-related images.

Therapy should focus not only on identifying the client's reactions to the illness, but also on her introjected images of women and femininity. In this way, she can explore the range of options permitted by her images. For some women, these images have emerged as a result of self-reflection, having been altered as circumstances demanded. These images of illness will be relatively malleable. For others, enculturated images have never been challenged. These women could be expected to have a greater struggle if their introjected images do not permit them the necessary flexibility to think, feel, and behave in ways that assist them in coping with cancer. As the constructs surrounding a client's perception of what it means to be a woman emerge, she can be invited to explore how her images of illness either facilitate or inhibit her recovery. One task of therapy is to separate a woman's experience from that of the enculturated dictums.

CONSTRUCTIVIST THERAPY TO ASSIST WOMEN IN COPING WITH CANCER

Deconstructing/Loosening Constructs. The process of deconstructing or loosening metaphors in therapy begins by immersing the client in the experience and allowing her an opportunity to focus on themes and metaphors. As the client fleshes out her own descriptions, she becomes aware of her idiosyncratic and sensory language, charged, colorful words, and figurative speech. Her ways of describing experiences and constructions of illness are then used to assist her in questioning her own introjected images. The process of heightening the client's awareness of her metaphors helps to move her away from broad stereotyped images and labels. As a result, her constructs loosen.

Lauren, a 43-year-old Euro-American construction foreperson, was diagnosed and undergoing treatment for advanced stages of breast cancer when she sought counseling. At one of her sessions she was in tears after yet another argument with her thirteen-year-old daughter that morning. Lauren remarked, "She won't let me be her mother; my cancer won't let me be her mother."

Of course, Lauren's true, underlying fear was that she would not "complete" her mothering role; its myriad ramifications were frequently the focus of therapy. However, for the purpose of this case illustration, we will focus on the cognitive aspects of Lauren's therapy. Her words also reflect a constructed image of "mother." Developmentally, how a woman defines herself in her mothering role changes as her children reach adolescence. However, Lauren's natural loosening of her constructs of mothering is complicated by her doubts in her ability to keep up her usual activities while fatigued from radiation treatments. Exploration of the experience of the argument with her daughter led to exploring her construction of "mother." She was then encouraged to explore her own underlying meaning associated with the construct of "mother." The process of bringing a construct into awareness, along with its supporting assumptions, results in loosening rigidly held constructs. As Lauren spoke about some of her assumptions, their absurdity in the current context became evident and she would laugh. Some parts of the original constructions of "mother" were easily dispelled by her. Other parts of the construct, however, required deeper exploration and reflection in order for her to determine whether they were important and should be retained.

The Origins of Construals. Another component of the deconstruction process is a mutual search for the genesis of the original images. This process occurs by focusing on how the constructs were learned. The process of adopting enculturated images and ideas occurs without critical thought. As she applies critical thinking to her constructs and their development, a client reappraises them such that the past legitimizes her experience by providing a rationale for how the construct developed. Not only does the content become legitimizing but also the process of choosing what she wants to retain is legitimizing and thus empowering. Providing an environment that allows for critical thinking results in the client experiencing her thoughts as legitimate and understandable, given her life history and cultural context. As a result of these insights and heightened awareness, she becomes more empowered and is able to see the impact that the cancer has on her life in a different, often less damaging light.

Lauren's construction of mother was "one who was *always* there for her children" and "one whose children's needs are fulfilled." Exploration of the components and origins of that construct led to a story from her own youth. At the young age of 14, Lauren was experiencing emotional pain associated with her far-from-ideal relationship with her neglectful, self-centered mother. It was at this point in her life that Lauren made a promise to herself to "always to be there for her children." It was at this point in Lauren's life that she began to build a construct of "mother" with all the wisdom and worldliness a hurt fourteen-year-old could muster. Naturally, her constructs included the rigidity common to a 14-year-old's moralistic way of judging as well. The construction emphasized those things that Lauren did not receive from her mother. Her construct of "mother" did not have the balance and flexibility necessary to guide her through her daughter's transition into adolescence in the face of her own illness and fear of death.

Co-Creating New Constructs. As a woman is encouraged to challenge her underlying assumptions, her own story emerges. This process, in itself, legitimizes her present feelings. From this new story, a woman will begin to revise her existing cognitive schemata (constructs). This new story, in turn, will result in new self-definitions, new options for acting, and empowerment to make behavioral changes. Carefully constructed new definitions for herself are then structured into a coherent schema that is capable of directing a larger range of behavior. Expanding the range of behavior inherent in a complex schemata, enhances the chances of new, more effective, behaviors being maintained and transferred.

The therapist assists the client in revising constructs or creating new ones by using the client's own idiosyncratic thoughts and sensory experiences. In the ongoing discourse, a client may use an analogy without realizing the impact. In one session, Lauren stated, "It's like I am a half dead chicken lying on the white line in the middle of the road, waiting for the next thing to hit me—roadkill!" This image led to a discussion about how she could save herself by moving out of the middle of the road.

Exploration of the meanings attached to the metaphor led to the development of a new, more proactive one. She decided that she would have to stand up and decide to which side of the road she would go. Further exploration of the meanings underlying this emerging image opens up new ways of thinking, new self-definitions, new assumptions, and ultimately new ways of acting. The new construct, a person who stands up and decides for herself, is more empowering than the "passive victim metaphor" that previously guided her response to cancer and cancer treatment.

As Lauren sorted through her underlying assumptions, she was encouraged to apply critical thought and determine which she would retain and which she would reject. Two of the assumptions Lauren rejected were "being there all the time" and "fulfilling my child's every need." In her exploration she recognized "listening to my child" was not part of the original construct, yet it was a quality she had grown to value. This alteration led Lauren to recognize she would not evaluate her mothering by whether she could coerce her daughter into eating a healthy breakfast or even if she could prepare breakfast when the fatigue from her illness overwhelmed her. She decided to judge herself on how well she listened to her daughter. At this point in her therapy, as new constructs are being built, Lauren would find difficulty releasing the moralistic component of her previous constructs. The new construct still retains some of the rigidity.

Enlarging the Scope of the Metaphor. The next step in the constructivist therapeutic process focuses on enlarging the range of behavior guided by the new construct. This is done by encouraging the client to become aware of other situations in which the empowered, decision-making person may act differently and be perceived differently. A construct becomes more accessible with use (Fazio, Blascovich, & Driscoll, 1992; Schuette & Fazio, 1995) and is likely to influence more areas of behavior. By evoking the construct directly, a person no longer has to think through each new behavior separately, which makes it more likely to generalize beyond the counseling session. Formulating a new construct in this manner actually creates a complex of behaviors that are then triggered by simply evoking the image or a new metaphor.

Further exploration of Lauren's newly-developed construct of "mother" led to discussions of specific situations, such as, "Could she always listen to her daughter?" At this point in the therapeutic process, the therapist initiates a discussion about the complex, often competing, roles experienced by women. In Lauren's case, these roles centered on her own needs for intimacy with her husband, the care of her other child, and swimming (Lauren's personal passion). By exploring each issue individually, Lauren was provided with the experience of maintaining flexibility and permeability in her newly-developing construct of "mother." That is, her construct was revised repeatedly. This process is complex, given that constructs are organized into a larger schema in which they overlap; for instance, her construct of "mother" also overlapped with her construct of "woman," and of "cancer patient," and of "wife."

The process of exploring, altering, and adapting constructs is conducted through the exploration of deeply personal idiosyncratic events that have formulated these constructs. The process often strips away the framework and the client is faced with exploring the raw emotional experience that led to the development of that construct. Lauren cried over the neglect experienced in her childhood until she reached resolution and forgave her mother. She cried over the enormous threat of dying before her children were grown. She cried over the impact on her intimacy with her husband the cancer had wrought.

Creating a Referent Group. The process of co-constructing new metaphors is creative, pro-active, and inherently social. Because constructs are created within a social interaction, they must also be maintained within a social interaction. This is one reason why support groups have been so effective in promoting changes in health behaviors and coping among cancer patients (Bloom & Spiegel, 1984; Fawzy et al., 1993; Fawzy et al., 1990; Spiegel,

Bloom, Kraemer, & Gottheil, 1989). This is also why a referent group is critical to the re-appraisal process necessary for effective coping (Leventhal et al., 1986; Rodin, 1978). Another way is using Michael White's concept of creating an audience (White, 1991) to establish a referent group. White suggests that in order for a behavior to become part of one's repertoire it must have the support of someone else. The thought of that person(s) is invoked whenever the behavior is considered.

Lauren was a quiet, private woman. She described herself as "not a joiner." Therefore she had no interest in a support group. Adapting Michael White's strategy of creating an audience, Lauren created her own support network. Through more intimate sharing with her husband Lauren re-established and deepened their intimacy. Lauren's trust and openness with a friend of many years was also strengthened. Lauren reconnected with female friends who, in the past, had served as distractions when she needed an escape from her personal struggles. Lauren created the network of support she needed to maintain her new constructs as her daughter sought her own independence, as her energy ebbed and flowed, despite Lauren's mother continuing to behave in well-entrenched patterns.

Maintaining the Sense of Empowerment. The sense of empowerment is maintained through the changes in a client's constructs. By treating a person's constructs as guides rather than reified truths, a client gains the ability and permission to scrutinize constructs as they no longer serve their purpose, thus increasing flexibility of behavior. This leads to increased flexibility in the woman's behavioral repertoire. She learns to allow new information to permeate the constructs, thus increasing their adaptability to new situations. She also experiences a greater sense of control knowing that her constructs are her own and she has the ability to change them when they no longer fit the context. She learns to use constructs within a certain range of situations that can be expanded or shrunk. This allows the constructs not only to change but also to be subjected to re-prioritization when necessary.

Concomitant with internalizing constructs of her own creation is a shift in perception toward a sense of control over life events. Belief in the controllability over life events leads to the use of more effective problem-solving and positive reappraisal and social support (Hilton, 1989), all of which have been associated with improved health outcomes (Altmaier, Lehman, Russell et al., 1992; Dunkel-Schetter, Feinstein, Taylor, & Falke, 1994; James, Thorn, & Williams, 1993).

CONCLUSION

A social constructivist method of conducting therapy with women who have been diagnosed with cancer is one viable method for remedying? revising? bludgeoning???!! existing illness metaphors. It is imperative that women reconstruct the meaning underlying their diagnosis in a way that will promote their emotional well-being. It will be no easy task to "exorcise the demon from the image of cancer" (Dagrosa, 1980, p. 326) given the lengthy and strong roots associated with existing medical metaphors. However, failure to attempt to facilitate a better understanding of these constructions and promote this shift could easily be construed as a form of "intellectual violence against women" (Bricker-Jenkins, 1994, p. 25). Such apathy is not acceptable. As Audre Lorde stated, "And where the words of women are crying to be heard, we must each of us recognize our responsibility to seek those words out, to read them and share them and examine them in their pertinence to our lives. That we not hide behind the mockeries of separations that have been imposed upon us and which so often we accept as our own" (Lorde, 1980, p. 23).

REFERENCES

Acterberg, J. (1990). *Woman as healer.* Boston: Shambala Press.

Adler, S. R., & Fosket, J. R. (1999). Disclosing complementary and alternative medicine use in the medical encounter: A qualitative study of women with breast cancer. *Journal of Family Practice, 48*(6), 453-458.

Albrecht, G., Walker, V., & Levy, J. (1982). Distance from the stigmatized: A test of two theories. *Science and Medicine, 16,* 1319-1327.

Altmaier, E.M., Lehman, T.R., Russell, D.W., & Weinstein, N. (1992). The effects of psychological interventions for rehabilitation of low back pain: A randomized, controlled trial evaluation. *Pain, 49*(3), 329-335.

Anderson, B. L., Anderson, B., & deProsse, C. (1989a). Controlled prospective longitudinal study of women with cancer. I. Sexual functioning outcomes. *Journal of Consulting and Clinical Psychology, 57*(6), 683-691.

Anderson, B. L., Anderson, B., & deProsse, C. (1989b). Controlled prospective longitudinal study of women with cancer. II. Psychological outcomes. *Journal of Consulting and Clinical Psychology, 57*(6), 692-697.

Anderson, B. L., & Jochimsen, P. R. (1985). Sexual functioning among breast cancer, gynecologic cancer, and healthy women. *Journal of Consulting and Clinical Psychology, 53*(1), 25-32.

Antonucci, T.C. (1985). Social support: Theoretical advances, recent findings, and pressing issues. In I.G. Sarason & B.R. Sarason (Eds.). *Social support: Theory, research, and applications* (pp. 21-49). Boston: Marinus Nyhoff Publishers.

Apfel, R. J., Love, S. M., & Kalinowski (1994). Keep abreast: Women and breast cancer in context. In M. P. Mirkin (Ed.), *Women in context: Toward a feminist reconstruction of psychotherapy* (pp. 217-236). New York: Guilford Press.

Banks & Kerns (1996). Explaining high rates of depression in chronic pain: A diathesis-stress framework. *Psychological Bulletin, 119,* 95-110.

Batt, S. (1994). *Patient no more.* Charlottetown, P.E.I., Canada: Gynergy Books.

Bauwens, E., & Anderson, S. (1993). Social and cultural influences on health care. In M. Stanhope & J. Lancaster (Eds.), *Community health nursing process and practice of promoting health (3rd edition, pp. 93-95).* St. Louis, MO: Mosby Yearbook.

Begbie, S. D., & Kersetes, Z. L. (1996). Patterns of alternative medicine by cancer patients. *Medical Journal of Australia, 165*(10), 545-548.

Berger, P.L., & Luckman, T. (1966). *The social construction of reality.* New York: Doubleday.

Betz, N. (1993). Women's career development. In F. L. Denmark & M. A. Paludi (Eds.), *Psychology of women: A handbook of issues and theories* (pp. 627-684). Westport, CT: Greenwood Press.

Bloom, J. R., Grazier, K., Hodge, F., & Hayes, W. (1991). Factors affecting the use of screening mammography among African American women. *Cancer Epidemiology, Biomarkers, and Prevention, 1,* 75-82.

Bloom, J. R., & Kessler, L. (1994). Emotional support following cancer: A test of the stigma and social activity hypothesis. *Journal of Health and Social Behavior, 35,* 118-133.

Bloom, J., & Spiegel, D. (1984). The effect of two dimensions of social support on the psychological well-being and social functioning of women with advanced breast cancer. *Social Science and Medicine, 19,* 831-837.

Brackett, C. D., & Powell, L. H. (1988). Psychosocial and physiological predictors of sudden cardiac death after healing of acute myocardial infarction. *American Journal of Cardiology, 61,* 979-983.

Bricker-Jenkins, M. (1994). Feminist practice and breast cancer: The patriarchy has claimed my right breast. *Social Work in Health Care, 19*(3/4), 17-42.

Brickman, P., Rabinowitz, V. C., Karuza, J., Jr., Coates, D., Cohn, E., & Kidder, L. (1982). Models of helping and coping. *American Psychologist, 37*(4), 368-384.

Brownmiller, S. (1975). *Against our will: Men, women, and rape.* New York: Simon & Schuster.

Burtle, V. (1983). Therapeutic anger in women. In L. B. Rosewater & L. E. A. Walker (Eds.), *Handbook of feminist therapy: Women's issues in psychotherapy* (pp. 71-80). New York: Springer Publishing Company.

Butler, S., Chalder, T., Ron, M., & Wessely, S. (1991). Cognitive behavior therapy in chronic fatigue syndrome. *Journal of Neurological Neurosurgical Psychiatry, 54,* 153-158.

Case, R. B., Moss, A. J., Case, N., McDermott, M., & Eberly, S. (1992). Living alone after myocardial infarction: Impact on prognosis. *Journal of the American Medical Association, 267* (4), 515-519.

Cassileth, B.R., Lusk, E.J., Strouse, T.B., & Miller, D.S. (1985). Psychosocial correlates of survival in advanced malignant disease. *New England Journal of Medicine, 312,* 1551-1555.

Conrad, P. (1980). On the medicalization of deviance and social control. In D. Ingleby (Ed.), *Critical psychiatry* (pp. 102-119). New York: Pantheon.

Cook, W. R. (1944, September). *The differential psychology of the American woman.* Presidential address given at the American Association of Obstetricians, Gynecologists and Abdominal Surgeons, 56th Annual Meeting, Hot Springs, VA.

Cooper, C. L., & Faragher, E. B. (1993). Psychosocial stress and breast cancer: The inter-relationship between stress events, coping strategies and personality. *Psychological Medicine, 23,* 653-662.

Cornwell, J. (1984). *Hard earned lives: Accounts of health and illness from East London.* London: Tavistock.

Dagrosa, T. W. (1980). Cancer in America: The socialization and promulgation of the mystique. *Nursing Forum, 19*(4), 324-334.

Datan, N. (1989). Illness and imagery: Feminist cognition, socialization, and gender identity. In M. Crawford & M. Gentry (Eds.), *Gender and thought: Psychological perspectives* (pp. 175-187). New York: Springer-Verlag.

Degner, L. F., Kristjansen, L. J., Bowman, D., Sloan, J. A., Carriere, K. C., O'Neil, J., Bilodeau, B., Watson, P., & Mueller, B. (1997). *Journal of the American Medical Association, 277*(18), 1485-1492.

Derogatis, L.R., Abeloff, M., & Melisaratos, N. (1979). Psychological coping mechanisms and survival time in metastatic breast cancer. *JAMA,* 242, 1504-1508.

Dimond, M. (1985). Social support and adaptation to chronic illness: The case of maintenance hemodialysis. *Research in Nursing and Health,* 2, 101-108.

Dobbin, J. P., Harth, M., McCain, G. A., Martin, R. A., & Cousin, K. (1991). Cytokine production and lymphocyte transformation during stress. *Brain, Behavior, and Immunity,* 5, 339-348.

Dunkel-Schetter, C., Feinstein, L.G., Taylor, S.E., & Falke, R.L. (1992). Patterns of coping with cancer. *Health Psychology,* 11(2), 79-87.

Epping-Jordan, J. E., Compas, B. E., & Howell, D. C. (1994). Predictors of cancer progression in young adult men and women: Avoidance, intrusive thoughts, and psychological symptoms. *Health Psychology, 13*(6), 539-547.

Esterling, B. A., Kiecolt-Glaser, J. K., Bodnar, J. C., & Glaser, R. (1994). Chronic stress, social support, and persistent alterations in the natural killer cell response to cytokines in older adults. *Health Psychology, 13*(4), 291-298.

Fawzy, F. I., Fawzy, N. W., Hyun, C. S., Elashoff, R., Guthrie, D., Fahey, J. L., & Morton, D.L. (1993). Malignant melanoma: Effects of early structured psychiatric intervention, coping, and affective states on recurrence and survival six years later. *Archives of General Psychiatry, 50,* 681-689.

Fawzy, F. I., Kemeny, M. E., Fawzy, N. W., Elashoff, R., Morton, D., Cousins, N., & Fahey, J. L. (1990). A structured psychiatric intervention for cancer patients: II. Changes over time in immunological measures. *Archives of General Psychiatry, 47,* 729-735.

Fazio, R. H., Blascovich, J., & Driscoll, D. M. (1992). On the functional value of attitudes: The influence of accessible attitudes on the ease and quality of decision making. *Journal of Personality and Social Psychology, 18*(4), 388-401.

Featherstone, C. (1996). Views of the body, stigma and the cancer patient experience. In A. Perry (Ed.), *Sociology: Insights in health care* (pp. 162-185). London: Arnold.

Ganz, P. A. (1998). Cancer: Medical aspects. In E. A. Blechman & K. D. Brownell (Eds.), *Behavioral medicine and women: A comprehensive handbook* (pp. 595-603). New York: The Guilford Press.

Geisser, M.E., Robinson, M.E., Keefe, F.J., & Weiner, M.L. (1994). Catastrophizing, depression, and the sensory, affective, and evaluative aspects of chronic pain. *Pain, 59*, 79-83.

Gillespie, R. (1995). The lay-professional encounter. In G. Moon (Ed.), *Society and health* (pp. 111-125). London: Routledge.

Goodwin, J. S., Hunt, W. D., & Samet, J. M. (1991). A population-based study of functional status and social support networks of elderly patients newly diagnosed with cancer. *Archives of Internal Medicine, 151*, 366-370.

Grann, V.R., Panageas, K.S., Antman, K.H., & Neugut, A.I. (1998). Decision analysis of prophylactic mastectomy and oophorectomy in BRCA1-positive or BRCA2-positive patients. *Journal of Clinical Oncology,* 16(3), 979-985.

Haber, S., Acuff, C., Ayers, L., Feeman, E. L., Goodheart, C., Kieffer, C. C., Lubin, L. B., Mikesell, S. G., Siegel, M., & Wainrib, B. C. (1995). Special populations: High-risk women, lesbian women, women of poverty and ethnicity, and older women. In (same authors) *Breast cancer: A psychological treatment manual* (pp. 61-70). New York: Springer Publishing Company.

Hafferty, F.W., & Light, D.W. (1995). Professional dynamics and the changing nature of medical work. *Journal of Health and Social Behavior,* Special No. Review, 132-53.

Heijmans, M., & deRitter, D. (1998). Assessing illness representations of chronic illness: Explorations of their disease-specific nature. *Journal of Behavioral Medicine,* 21(5), 485-503.

Heuser, L. (1991). Perceptions of women's emotional reactions to breast cancer. *SSR,* 75(4), 219-226.

Hilton, A. (1989). The relationship of uncertainty, control, commitment, and threat of recurrence to coping strategies used by women diagnosed with breast cancer. *Journal of Behavioral Medicine, 12*(1), 39-54.

Holland, J. C. (1991). Radiotherapy. In B. Fowble, R. L. Goodman, J. H. Glick, & E. F. Rosato (Eds.), *Breast cancer treatment: A comprehensive guide to management* (pp. 134- 145). Chicago, IL: Mosby Year Book.

Holland, J. C. (1992). Psychooncology: Where are we, and where are we going? *Journal of Psychosocial Oncology, 10*(2), 103-112.

Jensen, M.R. (1987). Psychobiological factors predicting the course of breast cancer. *Journal of Personality,* 55, 317-341.

Jones, E. E., Farina, A., Hastort, A. H., Markus, H., Miller, D. T., & Scott, R. A. (1984). *Social stigma.* San Francisco: Freeman.

Kaplan, H. S. (1992). A neglected issue: The sexual side effects of current treatments for breast cancer. *Journal of Sex & Marital Therapy, 18*(1), 3-19.

Keith, S. J. (1991). Surviving survivorship: Creating a balance. *Journal of Psychosocial Oncology, 9*(3), 109-115.

Keller, M., Henrich, G., Sellschopp, A., & Beutel, M. (1996). Between distress and support: Spouses of cancer patients. In L. Baider, C. L. Cooper, & A. deNour (Eds.), *Cancer and the family* (pp. 187-222). New York: John Wiley & Sons.

King, M.C., Powell, S., & Love, S.M. (1993). Inherited breast and ovarian cancer: What are the risks? What are the choices? *JAMA,* 269(15), 1975-1980.

Kreitler, S., Kreitler, H., & Shaked, T. (1997). Psychological and medical predictors of disease course in breast cancer: A prospective study. *European Journal of Personality, 11,* 383-400.

Lakoff, G., & Johnson, M. (1980). *Metaphors we live by.* Chicago: University of Chicago Press.

Langer, E. J., Chanowicz, B., Palmerino, M., Jacobs, S., Rhodes, M., & Thayer, P. (1990). Nonsequential development in aging. In C. Alexander & E. Langer (Eds.), *Higher stages of human development* (pp. 114-138). New York: Oxford University Press.

LaRossa, D. (1991). Reconstructive surgery. In B. Fowble, R. L. Goodman, J. H. Glick, & E. F. Rosato (Eds.), *Breast cancer treatment: A comprehensive guide to management* (pp. 311-324).Chicago, IL: Mosby Year Book.

Lerman, C., Biesecker, B., Benkendorf, J. L., Kerner, J., Gomez-Camino, A., Hughes, C., & Reed, M.M. (1997). Controlled trial of pretest education approaches to enhance informed decision making for BRCA 1 gene testing. *Journal of National Cancer Institute, 89*(2), 148-157.

Lerman, C., Daly, M., Walsh, W. P., Resch, N., Seay, J., Barsevick, A., Birenbaum, L., Heggan, T., & Martin, G. (1993). Communication between breast cancer and health care providers for patients' adjustment. *Cancer, 72,* 2612-2620.

Leventhal, H., Easterling, D.V., Coons, H., Luchterland, C., & Love, R.R. (1986). Adaptation to chemotherapy treatments. In B. Anderson (Ed.), *Women with cancer* (pp. 172-203). New York: Springer-Verlag.

Levy, S.M., Herberman, R.B., Whiteside, T., Sanzo, K., Lee, J., & Kirkwood, J. (1990). Perceived social support and tumor estrogen/progesterone receptor status as predictors of natural killer cell activity in breast cancer patients. *Psychosomatic Medicine, 52*(1), 73-85.

Lichtman, R. R., Taylor, S. E., & Wood, J. V. (1987). Social support and marital adjustment after breast cancer. *Journal of Psychosocial Oncology, 5*(3), 47-74.

Lorde, A. (1980). *The cancer journals.* San Francisco, CA: Aunt Lute Press.

Lupton, D. (1994). Femininity, responsibility, and the technological imperative: Discourses on breast cancer and the Australian press. *International Journal of Health Services, 24*(1), 73-89.

Lupton, D. (1995). Representations of medicine, illness and disease in elite and popular culture. In D. Lupton, *Medicine as culture: Illness, disease and the body in Western Societies* (pp. 50-78). Thousand Oaks, CA: Sage Publications.

MacKinnon, C. A. (1989). *Toward a feminist theory of the state.* Cambridge, MA: Harvard University Press.

Maturana, H., & Varella, F. (1987). *Tree of knowledge.* Boston: Shambala Press.

McBride, A. B. (1987). Position paper. In A. Eichler & D. L. Perron (Eds.), *Women's mental health: Agenda for research* (pp. 28-41). Rockville, MD: National Institute of Mental Health.

McCharen, N., & Earp, J. A. L. (1981). Toward a model of factors influencing the hiring of women with a history of breast cancer. *Journal of Sociology and Social Welfare, 8,* 346-363.

Morrison, V. (1992). Responding in a crisis: Perspectives on HIV, drugs, and women's needs in Edinburgh. In N. Dorn & S. Henderson (Eds.), *AIDS: Women drugs and social care* (pp. 30-50). London: Famer Press.

Nezu, A. M., Nezu, C. M., Friedman, S. H., Faddis, S., & Houts, P. S. (1999). *Helping cancer patients cope: A problem-solving approach.* Washington, DC: American Psychological Association.

Novack, D. H., Plumer, R., & Smith, R. L. (1979). Changes in physician's attitudes toward telling the cancer patient. *Journal of the American Medical Association, 24,* 897-900.

Noyes, R., & Kathol, R. G. (1986). Depression and cancer. *Psychiatric Developments, 2,* 77-100.

Oken, D. (1961). What to tell cancer patients: A study of medical attitudes. *Journal of the American Medical Association, 175,* 1120-1128.

Parker, I., Georgaca, E., Harper, D., McLaughlin, T., & Stowell-Smith, M. (1995). *Deconstructing psychopathology.* Thousand Oaks, CA: Sage Publications.

Parry, A., & Doan, R.E. (1994). *Story revisions.* New York: Guilford Press.

Parsons, T. (1972). Definitions of health and illness in light of American values and social structure. In E.G. Jaco (Ed.), *Patients, physicians, and illness* (2nd ed., pp. 107-127). New York: Free Press.

Pasacreta, J., McCorkle, R., & Margolis, G. (1991). Psychosocial aspects of breast cancer. In B. Fowble, R. L. Goodman, J. H. Glick, & E. F. Rosato (Eds.), *Breast cancer treatment: A comprehensive guide to management* (pp. 551- 570). Chicago, IL: Mosby Year Book.

Patterson, J. T. (1987). *The dread disease: Cancer and modern American culture.* Cambridge, MA: Harvard University Press.

Peters-Golden, H. (1982). Breast cancer: Varied perceptions of social support in the illness experience. *Social Science in Medicine, 16,* 483-491.

Petersen, S., Heesacker, M., & Marsh, R. (in press). Medical decision-making and coping among cancer patients. *Journal of Counseling Psychology.*

Petersen, S., Heesaker, M., Schwartz, S., & Marsh, R. (2000). Medical decision-making among cancer patients. *The Journal of Psychology & Health: An International Journal, 15,* 663-675.

Pettingale, K.W., Morris, T., Greer, S., & Haybrittle, J.L. (1985). Mental attitudes to cancer: An additional prognostic factor. *Lancet, 1,* 750.

Polomano, R. C., Hagopian, G. A., & McEvoy, M. D. (1991). Management of the effects of breast cancer therapy and progressive disease. In B. Fowble, R. L. Goodman, J. H. Glick, & E. F. Rosato (Eds.), *Breast cancer treatment: A comprehensive guide to management* (pp. 457-488). Chicago, IL: Mosby Year Book.

Power, P. (1979). The chronically ill husband and father: His role in the family. *The Family Coordinator, 2,* 616-621.

Radley, A., & Greene, R. (1986). Bearing illness: Study of couples where the husband awaits coronary graft surgery. *Social Science Medicine, 23,* 577-581.

Ray, C., Jefferies, S., & Weir, W.R.C. (1995). Coping and chronic fatigue syndrome: Illness responses and their relationship with fatigue, functional impairment, and emotional status. *Psychological Medicine, 25,* 937-945.

Rodin, J. (1978). Somatopsychics and attribution. *Personality and Social Psychology Bulletin, 4*(4), 531-540.

Rose, J. H. (1990). Social support and cancer: Adult patients' desire for support from family, friends, and health professionals. *American Journal of Community Psychology, 18,* 439-464.

Ruberman, W., Weinblatt, E., Goldberg, J. D., & Chaudharg, B.S. (1984). Psychosocial influences on mortality after myocardial infarction. *New England Journal of Medicine, 311,* 552-559.

Russo, N. F., & Denmark, F. L. (1984). Women, psychology and public policy: Selected issues. *American Psychologist, 39,* 1161-1165.

Sabo, D., Brown, J., & Smith, C. (1986). The male role and mastectomy: Support groups and men's adjustment. *Journal of Psychosocial Oncology, 4*(1/2), 19-31.

Scar, S., Phillips, D., & McCartey, K. (1989). Working mothers and their families. *American Psychologist, 44,* 1402-1409.

Scharfe, E., & Toole, S. (1992). HIV and the invisibility of women: Is there a need to redefine AIDS? *Feminist Review, 41,* 64-67.

Schuette, R. A., & Fazio, R. H. (1995). Attitude accessibility and motivation as determinants of biased processing: A test of the MODE model. *Journal of Personality and Social Psychology, 21*(7), 704-710.

Siegel, K. (1990). Psychosocial oncology research. *Social Work and Health Care, 15*(1), 21-43.

Smith, T.W., Christensen, A.J., Peck, J.R., & Ward, J.R. (1994). Cognitive distortion, helplessness, and depressed mood in rheumatoid arthritis: A four-year longitudinal analysis. *Health Psychology, 13*(3), 213-217.

Smith, N., & Reilly, G. (1994). Sexuality and body image: The challenge facing male and female cancer patients. *Canadian Journal of Human Sexuality, 3*(2), 145-149.

Sontag, S. (1989). *Illness as metaphor.* London: Penguin Press.

Spiegel, D. (1995). Social support and cancer. In N.R.S. Hall-Faltman, & S.J. Blumenthal (Eds.). Mind-body interactions and disease. Rockville, MD: Health.

Spiegel, D., Bloom, J. R., Kraemer, H. C., & Gottheil, E. (1989). Effect of psychosocial treatment on survival of patients with metastatic breast cancer. *The Lancet, 2,* 888-889.

Stacey, M. (1994). Feminist reflections on the General Medical Council: Recreation and retention of male power. In S. Wilkinson & C. Kitzinger (Eds.), *Women and health: Feminist perspectives* (pp. 181-202). New York: Taylor & Frances.

Stahly, G. B. (1988). Psychosocial aspects of the stigma of cancer: An overview. *Journal of Psychosocial Medicine, 6,* 3-4.

Stefanek, M. E., Shaw, A., DeGeorge, D., & Tsottles, N. (1989). Illness-related worry among cancer patients: Prevalence, severity, and content. *Cancer Investigations, 7*(4), 365-371.

Stetz, K.M., Lewis, F.M., & Primono, J. (1988). Family coping strategies and chronic illness in the mother. *Family Relations, 35,* 515-522.

Temoshek, L. (1985). Biopsychosocial studies on cutaneous malignant melanoma: Psychosocial factors associated with prognostic indicators, progression, psychophysiology, and tumor-host response. *Social Science and Medicine, 20,* 883-840.

Thompson, S. C., & Fitts, J. S. (1992). In sickness and in health: Chronic illness, marriage, and spousal caregiving. In S. Spacapan & S. Oskamp (Eds.), *Helping and being helped: Naturalistic studies* (pp. 115-151). Newbury Park, CA: Sage Publications.

Turk, D.C., Rudy, T.E. & Salovey, P. (1986). Implicit models of illness. *Journal of Behavioral Medicine, 9*, 453-474.

Turner, B. S. (1995). Professions, knowledge, and power. In B. S. Turner, *Medical power and social knowledge* (2nd ed., pp. 129-152). Thousand Oaks, CA: Sage Publications.

Waltz, M. (1986). Marital context and post-infarction quality of life: Is it social support or something more? *Social Science Medicine, 22*(8), 791-805.

Waxler-Morrison, N., Hislop, T. G., Mears, B., & Kan, L. (1991). Effects of social relationships on survival for women with breast cancer: A prospective study. *Social Science & Medicine, 33*, 177-183.

Weiner, B., Perry, R. P., & Magnusson, J. (1988). An attributional analysis of reactions to stigmas. *Journal of Personality and Social Psychology, 55*(5), 738-748.

Weitzman, L. M., & Fitzgeral, L. F. (1993). Employed mothers: Labor force profiles and diverse lifestyles. In J. Frankel (Ed.), *Employed mothers and the family context*. New York: Springer.

White, M. (1991). Deconstruction and therapy. *Dulwich Centre Newsletter, 3*, 21-40.

Wilkinson, S., & Kitzinger, C. (1994). Toward a feminist approach to breast cancer. In S. Wilkinson & C. Kitzinger (Eds.), *Women and health: Feminist perspectives* (pp. 124-140). New York: Taylor & Frances.

Worden, W., & Weisman, D. (1988). The emotional impact of recurrent cancer. *Journal of Psychosocial Oncology*, Win., *3*(4), 5-16.

Worell, J., & Remer, P. (1992). Changing roles for women. In J. Worell & P. Remer *Feminist perspectives in therapy: An empowerment model for women* (pp. 26-53). New York: John Wiley & Sons.

Putting Theory into Practice:
A Psychologist's Story

Pamela C. Fischer

SUMMARY. A diagnosis of breast cancer is a frightening and life-changing experience. It affects not only the physical body, but also one's psychological well-being and basic assumptions about the world. Paradoxically, having breast cancer can provide an opportunity for personal growth and finding new meaning in life. While coping with cancer is basically an individual task, coping skills, social support, and an empathic therapist can help the breast cancer patient manage this stressful time. This article explores my own experience with breast cancer and the resources and coping strategies that were most helpful in getting through this frightening time. I will discuss how my experience forced me to face my own mortality and led me to an inner strength and courage that I had not used before. By joining the ranks of those who have faced intense anxiety and fear during a serious life crisis, I have greater empathy for and understanding of my own patients' struggles.

Pamela C. Fischer, PhD, is a psychologist at the Department of Veterans Affairs Medical Center in Oklahoma City. She is also Assistant Clinical Professor in the Department of Psychiatry and Behavioral Sciences at Oklahoma University Health Sciences Center and Adjunct Professor in the Department of Psychology at Oklahoma City University. The use of the word patient instead of client throughout the article reflects only the setting in which she works the majority of the time. Dr. Fischer has a small private practice where she sees clients.

The author would like to thank Dr. Ellyn Kaschak for her helpful comments and willingness to mentor a first time contributor. She does indeed put theory into practice.

Address correspondence to: Pamela C. Fischer, Dept. of Veterans Affairs Medical Center, Psychology Service #183A, 921 N.E. 13th Street, Oklahoma City, OK 73104 (E-mail: Pamela.Fischer@med.va.gov).

[Haworth co-indexing entry note]: "Putting Theory into Practice: A Psychologist's Story." Fischer, Pamela C. Co-published simultaneously in *Women & Therapy* (The Haworth Press, Inc.) Vol. 23, No. 1, 2001, pp. 101-109; and: *Minding the Body: Psychotherapy in Cases of Chronic and Life-Threatening Illness* (ed: Ellyn Kaschak) The Haworth Press, Inc., 2001, pp. 101-109. Single or multiple copies of this article are available for a fee from The Haworth Document Delivery Service [1-800-342-9678, 9:00 a.m. - 5:00 p.m. (EST). E-mail address: getinfo@haworthpressinc.com].

KEYWORDS. Breast cancer, psychological well-being, personal growth, coping

As a psychologist, I work with individuals who are attempting to cope with a life trauma. Some are facing immediate crises, while others are trying to resolve issues from traumatic events that occurred years ago. Survivors of the Murrah Building bombing, the devastating Oklahoma tornado that took lives and leveled houses in May, 1999, combat veterans of the Viet Nam war, and others facing personal losses are my patients. Because I teach coping skills and help people work through trauma, some might assume that I could easily cope with whatever came my way. That assumption would be wrong.

Being diagnosed with breast cancer at the age of 47 was such an experience for me. That diagnosis raised a multitude of physical and emotional issues. In a matter of minutes, life changed. Beliefs and expectations about the future and about being a woman were suddenly challenged. Being diagnosed with this disease is not unusual. One out of eight women in the United States has breast cancer. However, as a psychologist with breast cancer, I now had a unique opportunity to practice those coping skills that I teach others. Instead of providing support, I was the one now looking to others for strength and encouragement and I was to find an inner strength and courage I had not used before.

A suspicious mass detected in a routine mammogram was the beginning of my ordeal with breast cancer. Instead of the standard "Everything looks normal" that I expected to hear from my radiologist, I was told to "find yourself a surgeon." Those words put into motion an anxiety I have not often felt in my life. Even though I had been unknowingly living with the tumor, at least for a few months, I became overcome with an urgency to get it removed. In a panic, I began my search for a breast surgeon. Luckily, I found an excellent surgeon who worked me into his schedule and removed the tumor the next day in his office. Two days later the pathology report confirmed what the doctor suspected. I had breast cancer.

I recall feeling shocked, numb, and in a state of disbelief. How could I feel absolutely fine and at the same time have a life-threatening disease? How could something so small and evasive have such apocalyptic consequences? The cruel nature of this disease is that it grows silently within a healthy body, giving the recipient no indication of its lethal existence. In trying to come to terms with this inconsistency, I vacillated between disbelief and reality. There must be some mistake. Yet the fear that remained constant in the pit of my stomach reminded me it was not a mistake. My identity as a healthy, fit, middle-age woman was suddenly transformed into a patient facing a life-threatening disease. I began cleaning out closets (so someone else didn't have to do it) and trying to tell my daughters where all the Christmas decorations and keepsakes were stored.

During this emotional upheaval, when my world seemed to be falling apart, I had to make many life-changing decisions. It is ironic that at a time when you function on "automatic" and your mind is in a fog, you must make decisions that will determine the quality of your life forever. To make informed decisions, I had to become educated about things I had never even thought about. What is the best treatment for my type and size of cancer? What are the advantages of lumpectomy, partial or radical mastectomy, chemotherapy, radiation or a combination of the above? What types of reconstruction are available and do I want reconstruction? If I choose implants should they be filled with saline or silicone or should I forget implants and use my own tissue in a tram flap procedure? What is a tram flap procedure? The information-gathering process took on a literature review quality equal to that of preparing to write a dissertation. It was like the frantic cramming one does in clinical training to find out how to treat a patient with a disorder one has never encountered.

I went through a conservative process in my treatment called "staging." Therefore, my initial diagnosis and surgery lasted from November until the end of January. After the tumor was removed in the doctor's office and malignancy confirmed, additional breast tissue and lymph nodes were removed three weeks later. Another month later I went through a bilateral mastectomy and reconstruction. The benefit of staging is that it utilizes the most conservative treatment until more radical procedures are proven necessary. In addition, the patient is informed every step of the way (no more waking up without a breast as in the old days). The disadvantage to staging is that it can take several weeks. When people find out you are back in the hospital for more surgery they begin to assume that you are dying, which leads to more inquiries and unwanted explanations.

Whether one has a lumpectomy or a mastectomy, the body is no longer the same. There are physical changes that affect appearance and biological changes that affect body functions. Body image, "the image of the body that a person sees with the mind's eye . . . the psychological space where body, mind, and culture come together" (Hutchinson, 1994, p. 153) is drastically altered. Because Western culture places such value on the way a woman's body looks, particularly her breasts, accepting and adjusting to a body that feels, looks, and performs differently is not an easy task. "Everything about our socialization as females in a patriarchal culture leads us to value our selves in terms of our bodies—as objects of love, as childbearers, as nurturers, and as ornaments for men" (Hutchinson, 1994, p. 153). Intellectually, a woman may know that her value as a person is not about her body shape. However, deeply embedded messages about what is feminine, attractive, and sensual are difficult to completely erase.

In a recent study researchers found that body image was only of moderate concern to women with early stage breast cancer during the first year post surgery. Strongest concerns were the possibility of recurrence, premature death, pain, harm from adjuvant therapy, and overwhelming bills (Spencer, Lehman, Wynings, Arena, Carver, Antoni, Derhagopian, Ironson, & Love, 1999). This may reflect a change in women's attitudes about their bodies or imply that when confronted with having a life-threatening illness, body concerns become much less significant.

Despite the chaos and confusion, my over-riding goal was clear. I wanted to live and to do whatever was necessary to give me the best chance of having that happen. My second goal was to continue my life as normally as possible. Though I have never been a person who relied on my body shape to form my identity, it became very important for me to look as much like my old self as possible. Looking the same would give the outward impression that I was the same. I could convince myself as well as others that my life would continue as normal.

Between surgeries I continued to work at the medical center and in my own private practice seeing patients in individual and group psychotherapy. Working kept me focused in other directions and, for the most part, allowed me to concentrate on the patient's world and temporarily forget my own. I did not tell my patients about my medical condition, concerned they would try to take care of me. While I can now tell my story when it is in the interest of the patient to do so, at the time of my diagnosis and treatment, my emotions were too close to the surface. Talking about it could give way to emotions that would unfairly burden the patient. I did not have formal psychological help during this time, primarily because "informal" psychological help was readily available from supportive colleagues who let me take the lead. If I needed to talk, I could. Otherwise, no one pressured me for the latest details.

Staying busy with work and family helped me keep my anxiety to a manageable level, although the idea of having cancer never left my mind. However, there were unpredictable times when I would become so anxious that I had to take some action to relieve it. I remember standing in the cafeteria line chatting with a co-worker, when suddenly I became so anxious that I had to leave. Walking back to my office and up eight flights of stairs helped calm me. Deep breathing, positive affirmations, and calming self-talk became part of my daily routine, as did cognitive therapy techniques of challenging my catastrophic thinking.

Social support was extremely important to me during this time. I cannot imagine having to experience this alone. Friends can distract you with their stories and help keep your experience in perspective. Support groups that consist of women who have "been there" can be invaluable. I was fortunate to have a supportive spouse who served as an outlet for my fears when anxiety would soar. I also had patient-centered doctors who took the time to answer questions, suggest reading material, and put me in contact with women who had undergone the treatments I was considering.

I certainly grew in my spiritual life. Facing my own mortality caused me to take a long, hard look at life. I questioned whether I was spending time doing what I really want to do. Did my life have meaning? Was I taking the time to be the kind of mother, wife, psychologist and friend I wanted to be? Was I taking the time to enjoy life? The existential philosophers believe we can understand what it means to live only when we confront the possibility of our own death (Nauman, 1972). I found truth in this philosophy. Although I had encouraged people in therapy to look at their own lives and seek a balance, I had not necessarily applied that to my own life. My life centered predominately on a work ethic which left little time for relaxation and fun.

Journal keeping was an important activity for me. Daily I recorded my thoughts and feelings. Not only did writing help me vent my fears; it also proved to be a means of developing understanding and acceptance of my situation. Smyth and Pennebaker (1999) suggest that translating emotions about the event into words changes the way one organizes and thinks about the event. Thus, writing about a traumatic experience helps one cognitively process the event and assimilate it into one's schemas (Anderson, 1985; Fiske & Taylor, 1984) or basic assumptions about the world.

I went through a short, but agonizing period of blaming myself. Because we live in a society founded on the assumption that we can control our own destiny, when diagnosed with a disease, we want to know why and question what we did to cause the illness. A belief in the causal role of personality in the development of breast cancer is widespread, even among breast cancer patients (McKenna, Zevon, & Rounds, 1999). A number of theories about the connection between personality and breast cancer appear in the literature. For example, research indicates that breast cancer patients (a) experience heightened feelings of anxiety and depression (Cheang & Cooper, 1985); (b) have a conflict-avoidant personality style (Cooper, Davies-Cooper, & Braragher, 1986); (c) have difficulty expressing anger (Jansen & Muentz, 1984); and (d) use denial and repression as a psychological defense (Sherg, Cramer, & Blohmke, 1981).

I obsessed over whether drinking wine on the weekends increased my estrogen level and caused the development of my cancer and whether I had been too expressive of my emotions or not expressive enough. While I believe strongly in a mind-body connection, the notion that some aspect of my personality contributed to my having cancer ultimately seems to be a modern version of holding women responsible for any misfortune that befalls them. Self-blame is associated with increased symptoms of psychological distress (Glinder & Compas, 1999). If women do not feel depressed, anxious, and at least in part responsible for their diagnosis of cancer, they are more likely to take this issue into the political arena and press for the allocation of research resources. As Kathy LeTour (2000), a breast cancer survivor and journalist said, "There is a cure for breast cancer and it is called money."

Even though I have tried to integrate my experience into my professional life, I can not offer a definite set of guidelines or rules for counseling a woman diagnosed with breast cancer. The stage of cancer and type of treatment required bring different concerns, as does the age and life situation of the patient. However, my own concerns and fears about dying and leaving my family, choosing the best types of treatment, and adjusting to a different body physically and emotionally are relatively common among cancer patients. So is living with the insidious fear of reoccurrence.

From my own experience as patient and psychologist, what can I offer that could be helpful to someone treating a breast cancer patient? Basically, having cancer is a painful and lonely journey. While the support from family, friends, and professionals is invaluable, facing the possibility of one's own death is something one does alone. Thus, the major task of the therapist treating a patient in the initial stages of diagnosis is simply to provide a safe, holding environment (Winnicot, 1965). "A simple presence, accompanied by simple acceptance of what the other person is saying is enough" (Tedeschi & Calhoun, 1995, p. 103). Because the essence of the therapeutic relationship is based on empathy, "the capacity to participate in or experience another's sensations, feelings, thoughts or movements" (Havens, 1986), the therapist must be willing to open herself to the subjective experience of the patient and follow wherever she leads.

Hope is a necessary coping tool for surviving the cancer experience and has been shown to boost the immune system, increase the length of survival, and even change the course of the disease (Hafen, Karren, Frandsen, & Smith, 1996). Not until my diagnosis did I become aware how often cancer is still considered a death sentence. One need only to watch television to see that the cancer patient rarely survives. While the diagnosis of cancer does not carry the stigma it once did and the treatments for breast cancer are now more promising than ever, the word *cancer* still causes discomfort and distress among some with whom you associate. They seem to handle this distress by either avoidance or sharing cancer stories about others, not all of which have happy endings. At a time when anxiety is high and logical thinking is difficult to maintain, it is easy to take on another's story as your own and assume the worst. One of my colleagues helped me put this into perspective when he suggested that I had become a Rorschach for others who projected their own fears onto me. The therapist can provide a reality check for the patient and by doing so decrease anxiety and increase hope and optimism.

There is a fundamental sadness that accompanies the loss of bodily sensation and function. While there is clearly joy in being alive, there is unavoidable grief and longing for the way one used to be. Changes in reproductive capacity or being thrust into early menopause are often unexpected side effects of breast cancer treatment. Undergoing chemotherapy creates concerns about the adverse effect it may have on feelings of femininity, sexual desirability and capacity for sexual feelings (Spencer et al., 1999). Adjusting to and making peace with these changes is not an easy task. If the therapist has successfully negotiated similar changes in her life, self-disclosure can be a powerful source of reassurance and hope for the client.

The therapist can be a resource for helping the family adjust to this new situation if necessary. A diagnosis of cancer affects families, not just individuals. Family members may have difficulty accepting the diagnosis and be overwhelmed with conflicting feelings such as fear and sadness about the potential loss of a wife, mother, daughter or sister and anger that things are different. The quality of the relationships before diagnosis and the stability of the family will influence the adjustment of the family and the type of support they are able to provide.

After the emotional intensity of diagnosis and treatment passed and life was beginning to feel normal again, I began to try to make sense of my experience. How did being a cancer patient fit into my perception of myself as a woman and my beliefs and expectations about the world? How could I use this experience as a vehicle for growth? The frightening and negative aspects of having breast cancer are obvious, but what were the aspects of this experience that could be positive?

If we perceive life problems as teachers, as I often say in my therapy groups, then times of crisis are also opportunities for learning and growth. What did this disease teach me? My life is filled with wonderful people, meaningful work and pleasurable moments that I do not take time often enough to enjoy. Cancer forced me to confront my own mortality, which, in turn, caused me to realize how much I loved being alive. Tedeschi and Calhoun (1995) propose that a common element in the positive changes wrought by traumatic events is the appreciation of paradox. My experience with cancer was the loneliest time of my life. It was also a time when I felt the most loved and supported by others.

I believe that having cancer has made me more sensitive to others, heightened my sense of compassion, and made it possible for me to have more empathy with and understanding of my patients. It has also confirmed the notion that regardless of the precautions we take, there are things in life we cannot control. Learning to accept life as it is, fair or unfair, is one of life's greatest challenges.

Can a therapist help a woman with breast cancer find some meaning, some benefit in her experience? From my own work with survivors of trauma, I have learned that some individuals can readily identify the benefits of their experience, while others have more difficulty perceiving a positive aspect of their experience. However, the therapist's empathy, caring and willingness to listen to the patient's account of her struggle allow her to realize that her story is comprehensible and meaningful. This therapeutic connection can encourage her to perceive the *benefits* of her experience with cancer and develop a more profound sense of herself and the world. Through this process the breast cancer patient can become aware of her resilience, strength, and courage. Ultimately, however, and much like the personal course of the disease itself, the struggle to accept, understand and create meaning from having breast cancer is an individual process. It is a journey that each patient must make alone. The therapist can go only part of the way.

REFERENCES

Anderson, J. R. (1985). *Cognitive psychology and its implications* (2nd ed.), New York: Freeman.

Cheang, A., & Cooper, C. L. (1985). Psychosocial factors in breast cancer. *Stress Medicine, 1*, 61-66.

Cooper, C. L., Davies-Cooper, R. F., & Faragher, E. B. (1986). A prospective study of the relationship between breast cancer and life events, Type A behavior, social support and coping skills. *Stress Medicine, 2*, 271-277.

Fiske, S. T., & Taylor, S. E. (1984). *Social cognition.* Reading, MA: Addison-Wesley.

Glinder, J. G., & Compas, B. E. (1999). Self-blame attributions in women with newly diagnosed breast cancer: A prospective study of psychological adjustment. *Health Psychology, 18*, 475-481.

Hafen, B. Q., Karren, K. J., Frandsen, K. J., & Smith, N. L. (1996). *Mind/Body health.* Needham Heights, MA: Allyn & Bacon.

Havens, L. (1986). *Making contact: Uses of language in psychotherapy.* Cambridge, MA: University.

Hutchinson, M. A. (1994). Imagining ourselves whole: A feminist approach to treating body image disorders. In P. Fallon, M. Katzman, & S. Wooley (Eds.), *Feminist perspectives on eating disorders* (p. 153). New York: Guilford.

Jansen, M.A., & Muenz, L.R. (1984). A retrospective study of personality variables associated with fibrocystic disease and breast cancer. *Journal of Psychosomatic Research, 28*, 35-42.

Latour, K. (2000, May). Keynote address presented at the first meeting of the Project Woman Coalition Ribbons & Roses Annual Meeting, Oklahoma City, OK.

McKenna, M. C., Zevon, M. A., Corn, B., & Rounds, J. (1999). Psychosocial factors and the development of breast cancer: A meta-analysis. *Health Psychology, 18,* 520-530.

Nauman, S.E. (1972). *The new dictionary of existentialism.* Secaucus, NJ: Citadel Press.

Scherg, H., Cramer, I., & Blohmke, M. (1981). Psychosocial factors and breast cancer: A critical reevaluation of established hypotheses. *Cancer Detection and Prevention, 4,* 165-171.

Smyth, J. M., & Pennebaker, J. W. (1999). Sharing one's story: Translating emotional experiences into words as a coping tool. In Snyder, C. R. (Ed.), *Coping: The psychology of what works* (pp. 70-89). New York: Oxford University.

Spencer, S. M., Lehman, J.M., Wynings, A. P., Carver, C. S., Antoni, M. H., Derha-gopian, R. P., Ironson, G., & Love, N. (1999). Concerns about breast cancer and relations to psychosocial well-being in a multiethnic sample of early-stage pa-tients. *Health Psychology, 18,* 159-168.

Tedeschi, R. G., & Calhoun, L. G. (1995). *Trauma & transformation: Growing in the aftermath of suffering* (p. 103). Thousand Oaks, CA: Sage.

Winnicott, D.W. (1965). *The maturational processes and the facilitating environ-ment.* New York: International University Press.

Feminist Psychotherapy in Cases
of Life-Threatening Illness

Denise Twohey

SUMMARY. In this article the author discusses therapeutic issues facing clients and psychotherapists who deal with life-threatening illnesses. She writes from the dual perspective of feminist client and psychotherapist, having recently undergone surgery for the removal of a malignant brain tumor. Numerous feminist therapeutic issues have emerged post-surgically including changed relationships, new boundaries, individual denial, altered sexuality and existential issues. Personal vignettes introduce each subsection, culminating in considerations for psychotherapists. Conclusions are then drawn. *[Article copies available for a fee from The Haworth Document Delivery Service: 1-800-342-9678. E-mail address: <getinfo@haworthpressinc.com> Website: <http://www.HaworthPress. com> © 2001 by The Haworth Press, Inc. All rights reserved.]*

KEYWORDS. Life-threatening illness, relationships, boundaries, denial, sexuality, existential

I am writing from the dual perspective of feminist therapist and client, meaning sometimes I will speak as a psychotherapist and sometimes as a

Denise Twohey, EdD, is Associate Professor, University of North Dakota. Address correspondence to: Department of Counseling, Box 8255, University Station, University of North Dakota, Grand Forks, ND 58202-8255.

The author wishes to acknowledge the faculty writing group led by Libby Rankin, PhD, at the University of North Dakota, and Mary Lee Nelson, PhD, from the University of Seattle for their encouragement and support during the preparation of this manuscript.

[Haworth co-indexing entry note]: "Feminist Psychotherapy in Cases of Life-Threatening Illness." Twohey, Denise. Co-published simultaneously in *Women & Therapy* (The Haworth Press, Inc.) Vol. 23, No. 1, 2001, pp. 111-120; and: *Minding the Body: Psychotherapy in Cases of Chronic and Life-Threatening Illness* (ed: Ellyn Kaschak) The Haworth Press, Inc., 2001, pp. 111-120. Single or multiple copies of this article are available for a fee from The Haworth Document Delivery Service [1-800-342-9678, 9:00 a.m. - 5:00 p.m. (EST). E-mail address: getinfo@haworthpressinc.com].

cancer patient. I have been diagnosed with ogiloastrocytoma, a malignant brain tumor about the size of an egg. The tumor has been surgically removed, but my prognosis is uncertain. As a result of the surgery, I also suffer from other residual disabilities.

Because of this cancerous tumor, I am aware of therapeutic issues that I had not previously considered. I am writing about these issues because I believe that clients with life-threatening illnesses are often overlooked. They are most certainly overlooked by clinicians who want to ignore the fearful topic of both their clients' and their own mortality. Additionally, they may slip through the cracks of most social service agencies.

In this article, personal vignettes will introduce each subsection, culminating in considerations for psychotherapists. Topics include: Changing relationships, boundaries, denial, sexuality and existential issues.

CHANGING RELATIONSHIPS

"Why is everyone avoiding me?" Patients with life-threatening illnesses may feel like they're playing tag, and they're perpetually "it." I could not understand why so many people at work seemed to be avoiding me until one of my doctoral students explained. She said my very presence was a constant reminder to her of her own mortality. She added that she and I were about the same age. The fact that she had recently adopted a young daughter made her feel all the more vulnerable. Another of my doctoral advisees was afraid to call me. He did not want to trouble me for letters of recommendation for a job, which he desperately needed to support himself and his daughter. He was a single parent. I was confronted by my department chair because these students were avoiding me.

And what about my friends? Recently, at my suggestion, a group of my closest colleagues read *Over My Head: A Doctor's Own Story of a Traumatic Brain Injury from the Inside Out* (Osborn, 1998). The book proved to be enormously helpful to me in the months after surgery. However, when we met, I sensed some awkwardness in our discussion. When we gathered again, at my insistence, to discuss the awkwardness, my friends told me I did not have to pretend to discuss a book to talk about my fears. I realize now that my fears seemed contagious. If I could have been quarantined, people would not have had to deal with fears about mortality, either mine or their own.

So what are my fears? I am worried about physical pain. And spiritual pain, too. I am worried about running out of energy and money. I am also concerned about occupational malaise. I am full of regrets about things I'll never be able to do again, and sorrow about relationships that did not materialize.

Sports were very much a part of my former life. Now I cannot ski, play tennis, or run, as I could. I had previously pictured myself pursuing these interests well into old age. Now, relationships with former sports partners are permanently altered. Although we have memories and shared history, we will no longer create new memories together, at least not sporting ones.

More important I am worried about my intellect, which for all practical purposes results in the loss of more relationships. I cannot keep up with my friends' conversations anymore. My brain seems to function much more slowly these days. Although some of that slowness may just be an inevitable sign of aging, it is still very frustrating when I cannot keep up with the conversation.

Clients with serious illnesses confront many losses, including the invisible losses of long term relationships. By invisible, I mean that with the onset of a serious illness, one becomes a new person. By new person I mean that the relational qualities for which one was once admired must be altered for both oneself and one's friends. For example, I used to be a good cook, but not anymore. I was also a competent conversationalist, but once again not anymore. These changes have had a reciprocal effect resulting in new relationships with everyone and everything in my past life.

What is the role of the feminist therapist? A good therapist, whether feminist or not, can help her client grieve. She could be grieving either actual or potential losses. Actual loss could mean, for example, the loss of independence because of being unable to drive. Potential loss could mean the loss of future career options. I am also referring to the loss of mental agility. The therapist can normalize her client's experience of constant loss. And just as importantly, she can help her grieve the loss of possibilities. By anticipating new potential losses that might occur, she can gently prepare her client to deal with them.

What is the specific role of the feminist therapist? Clients may feel embarrassed by their new dependent status. A feminist therapist can reassure her client by acknowledging that relationships are central to women's lives (Gilligan, 1982; Kaschak, 1992). A feminist therapist understands and verbally acknowledges that, without relationships, most women's lives would lack meaning.

BOUNDARIES

"I want to see your psychologist with you," said my sister. It was an ongoing argument between us; I felt perfectly able to talk to him myself, and resented my sister's insistence on accompanying me. The therapist noted that boundary issues seemed to be a concern in my family of origin. Although he was not necessarily a feminist, I felt very supported by him. I felt supported by how he treated me as a fellow (sic) psychologist and not just as a patient.

For a time, I was really in need of help. My whole family's boundaries became blurred. Now I no longer need so much help, but my family is used to paying very close attention to me, sometimes too much attention. For example, my parents took charge of all of my finances while I was ill, and when I began to recover I felt like a small child asking for her allowance. I also felt overly exposed. Having all of one's financial matters available for parental review feels like being naked. "Are they judging my expenditures?" I wondered.

Families react curiously to the news of life-threatening illness. One benefit in my family of origin has been the stronger feeling of love that I sense coming from them and that I feel toward them. My mother now says "I love you" almost every time we talk. This has had a reciprocal effect on me. It is the one good thing I can think of about having cancer.

"Where I stop and you begin" may not be so clear anymore in families where serious illness occurs. Care of the patient usually entails intense family involvement in situations where the patient is unable to act on her or his own behalf. Such situations can exacerbate pre-existing family boundary issues and result in the patient feeling smothered, disregarded or both.

What is the role of the therapist in all of this? Imagine that Edie Brickel, a currently popular songwriter, wrote these lyrics about psychotherapy:

> I want someone to follow
>
> Who doesn't lead the way
>
> I want someone to listen
>
> Who won't repeat what I say

I especially like the lines about "someone to follow, who doesn't lead the way." The lyrics suggest a paradox, which is very similar to the paradox inherent in feminist therapy, with its emphasis on egalitarian and non-hierarchical relationships. Feminist therapy strives to build a relationship based on mutual respect. It is a collaborative process in which the therapist and client mutually decide on the goals, direction and pace of therapy (Worell & Johnson, 1997).

Once an egalitarian and mutually respectful relationship has been established, the therapist might help the client to articulate the limits of what family members or friends can do. If those boundaries are not respected, the client will be uncomfortable, distempered, and perhaps less likely to heal.

DENIAL

"Wait, wait—don't tell me!" Can anyone make good choices about health care when her or his own life is at stake? My sister fears I might not be

making good choices. I regret to say that she may be right. I certainly do not go out of my way to seek out information on ogiloastrocytoma. I was reassured about this seemingly odd behavior by my oncologist. He told me that he had suffered from Hodgkins disease while in medical school and consequently knew less about it than almost any other disease.

One study, reported in an article in the *New Yorker* magazine (Gawande, 1999), found that although 64% of the general population thought they would like to select their own cancer treatment, only 12% of newly diagnosed cancer patients actually, when the opportunity presented itself, wanted to do so.

My sister and I often argued about how active a role I should take in my treatment. She was surprised by my seeming passivity. Frankly, I was surprised by it too. If this article were about anyone else, I would say they were in denial. But it is about me. So, although on one level I recognize my denial, on another level I cannot admit it, even to myself.

Denial works in strange ways. What is the right amount when dealing with cancer? I recognize that my life may end prematurely. I really do not know about the odds. Did I forget to ask? No. Medical science is inexact. The studies that have been done on my type of cancer were completed in the 1980's; my surgery was much later and more aggressive than those studied. Furthermore, I'm informed, no studies will be performed on my type of cancer with my specific type of treatment. So it is anybody's guess how long I will live. I could have a recurrence tomorrow, ten years from now or maybe never.

Several years ago I saw a video made by a man who was dying of cancer. He spoke to this issue of denial. He advised the physicians for whom the video was made, above all else, to keep hope alive for the patient. I was puzzled by the paradox. Surely he must have known that he was dying. How could hope be kept alive? But now I think I understand it. There is a very thin line between hope and despair. Having hope can create the will to live. After all, we are all dying; it is just a question of when. My feminist therapist may want to consider giving denial a valid place in my life.

SEXUALITY

"When could I have sex again?" Everybody seemed to ignore my questions. Did they think I wasn't serious? Maybe they simply assumed that I wouldn't want to have sex again, or worse yet, that no one would want me as a sexual partner. Maybe they were right. Maybe not.

I had doubts about both my physical attractiveness and my sexuality before surgery, but I did not usually seem to lack sexual partners, and at least I had some affirmation of my attractiveness. Now I have no sexual partners and wonder if this void in my life will ever be filled. Maybe I should just be glad for the close friendships that almost satisfy me. But almost is such a big word. I guess I am still waiting for that special someone, even though he has not shown up yet after almost 16 years since my divorce.

And now I have cancer.

The following poems capture my feelings quite well:

(O)

I have

    not

        made love

In

    four

        years

I think my vagina

Has

    Died

And gone to heaven.

PLEASE

resurrect me!

        (Unpublished, Anonymous)

Sex . . . is not fun anymore.

I haven't changed

But you have.

    I am asexual

Because I have a handicap.

You're afraid of me,

Why?

I am the same person,

Loving,

    giving,

        and sometimes

A pain in the ass

Like everyone!

Like normal people.

(Unpublished, Anonymous)

Last Christmas, my mother said she could understand why I wanted to do what normal people were doing. We were arguing about whether I would be "allowed" to go to Atlanta for New Year's Eve. I eventually told her that I was 49 years old and I would be making my own decision about Atlanta. But what really stung was the way she used the term "normal people."

Who are the normal people? And what are they doing? One thing that I imagine them doing is having good, healthy, sexual relationships. Even if they're not, I'm imagining they are. Whereas I, on the other hand, have grave doubts about my femininity and my sexuality.

It doesn't help that I feel so unattractive with this almost bald head. Why did the radiologist fail to inform me until I went in for the first treatment that my hair might not grow back? A year after treatment, it still is not back. My lawyer friends tell me this was a breach of informed consent. Did the radiologist really think that I would not return for treatment? "Oh, you can always comb it over" he said appeasingly. Did he really think that I could be so easily appeased? Or did he think that because I have cancer, I would have no interest in sex, sexuality, or my appearance?

Some people assume that cancer patients are asexual. However, refraining from sex and being asexual is not the same thing. Sexuality is changed by cancer. How? Well, first of all, if the patient is involved in a long-term relationship, he or she may lack the energy for sex. Desire may very likely diminish while the patient is engaged in complex medical procedures. If the patient is not in a lasting relationship, she or he is unlikely to start one while dealing with a life-threatening illness (A. Lamson, personal communication, February 19, 1999).

Most people have difficulty discussing sex. This difficulty applies equally to the therapist and client with a life-threatening illness. Raising the topic may seem awkward at first, but once introduced can reap surprising benefits for the client.

The client may have internalized the outside world's reaction to her new "asexual" status. If the feminist therapist does not challenge her, she may believe she is really not interested in sex. Or alternately, she may really not see sexuality as a priority, in which case the therapist should follow her lead. I realize that I am presenting you with a contradiction. But that is where your clinical judgment comes in to play.

Feminist therapy works collaboratively with the client to challenge societal presumptions. A feminist therapist, above all, helps the client to create her own perspective, a perspective potentially fraught with contradictions, but nevertheless, her own (Worrell & Johnson, 1997).

EXISTENTIAL ISSUES

"You will die in my hands. You could live for two years, you could live for five years, maybe even ten, but you will eventually die in my hands." This was the message from one of the only two local neurosurgeons. In his statement, I heard notice that the power to influence my own fate was no longer mine. His words had a strange effect on me. I felt oddly mobilized, fueled by fury at his arrogance. Almost before he finished the sentence, I was asking for a second opinion. Not long after that I was hospitalized at the Mayo Clinic to await surgery by a different neurosurgeon.

Interestingly, my good friend who had been with me throughout the diagnostic phase of this ordeal was frightened by the initial neurosurgeon's words. In reconstructing our discussion, which we did before and during the preparation of this manuscript, she relived the same fears. She asked why I was not feeling, or at least not showing, similar emotions.

Maybe I felt like we were discussing ancient history. In other words, maybe I was finished with those emotions. Or maybe I was experiencing denial, again. However, I prefer to think that I had worked through whatever my friend thought I should be feeling. Let me describe for you when I think that happened.

One night at the Mayo Clinic, I was in an unbelievable amount of pain. My whole body had developed a rash which I could not keep from scratching. The nurse came in every hour to offer me Benedryl, which I had already ascertained did not work to relieve the pain. It sounds melodramatic, but I saw death as the only alternative to my pain.

I am embarrassed to say that previously I had always believed that I could either take or leave this life. The afterlife, however, promised to be an exciting mystery or a welcome reprieve, depending on my mood. That night, during which I did not sleep a wink, I wanted nothing more than to get out of this life and to gain admission to the next, that is, if there is an afterlife. If not, I still wanted out.

The next night I talked on the telephone with my mother. Somehow while I was talking with her, I realized that it was very selfish to desire death. I thought of all the pain my mother had endured (giving birth to five babies, for example). Eventually, that night, I turned a corner. I found that I was more attached to this life than I had previously believed. I really think that if I had not recommitted on that particular evening, during which I ended up in intensive care, I would not have gotten better at all.

How should a therapist talk about death with a client who may be terminally ill? First, he or she must have confronted her or his own fears about death and dying. I cannot think of any quick advice on how to do that, or even a way to guarantee that the task has been accomplished. Although I realize I may be contradicting myself, I think facing death is like shifting sand. One day you think you are all right with it. The next day you are not. Since I am possibly denying the timing of my own death, I am on very shaky ground here.

What if the death of your client is imminent? In a study involving 28 resident physicians working with dying patients, most of their encounters fell short of "working toward a good death" (Dozor & Addison, 1992). Of 30 stories about dying patients, only two were identified by these authors as "good deaths." What constitutes a good death? According to Dozor and Addison (1992) among other characteristics, a good death is characterized by (a) acceptance of mortality, (b) closeness, (c) intimacy, and (d) closure. Some actions taken by the residents to promote good deaths were (a) asking other residents for help, (b) addressing personal feelings, (c) involving the patient in conversations about illness and feelings, (d) touching the patient, (e) encouraging family to talk, etc. All of this advice is good for feminist therapists.

A feminist viewpoint can contribute to strengthening a client's understanding about how to maintain a sense of personal power, even when her health seems out of control. Small choices mean a lot. While hospitalized, even a choice about the menu can be meaningful, if it is one of the few choices the client feels she has left to her. Larger choices, like the decision about treatment options, can be very difficult, partly because they may be the last choices a client can exercise. A feminist therapist, by virtue of being outside of the immediate family, may be better able to help the patient work through these options.

CONCLUSIONS

In this brief article I have examined many poignant issues for the patient with a life threatening illness. To summarize, I would point out that relationships may be changing for her. In fact, every single relationship she has with persons, with things, or with ideas, is entirely new to her. I cannot emphasize enough the need for sensitivity of the therapist, in helping her or his client manage these sometimes startling, sometimes subtle, changes.

Former friends might react oddly to her new status. They may avoid her, smother her, ignore her or alternate among all three. Boundaries may be blurred. She may feel disregarded by both family and friends. However, as I've said above, their avoidance of her may be more about their own fears of mortality than about hers.

The client may deny the seriousness of her situation. The good feminist

therapist will not necessarily confront her. When and if he or she does challenge her, they must pay very close attention to timing of any confrontation in
order to be respectful of the client's timeline.

Whether she has experienced radiation, chemotherapy or some other form
of treatment, her sense of self may have changed dramatically. The client may
have concerns about her sexuality, femininity, and physical and psychological attractiveness. Lastly, she might have some important feelings about her
own death that it might help her to articulate.

REFERENCES

Dozer, R.B., & Addison, R.B. (1992). Toward a good death: An interpretive inves-
    tigation of family practice residents' practices with dying patients. *Family Medi-
    cine, 24*, 538-543.
Gawande, A. (1999, October). Whose body is it, anyway? *The New Yorker.*
Gilligan, C. (1982). *In a different voice.* Cambridge: Harvard University Press.
Kaschak, E. (1992). *Engendered lives.* New York: Basic Books.
Lamson, A. (February 19, 1999). Personal communication.
Osborn, C. (1998). *Over my head: A doctor's own story of traumatic brain injury
    from the inside looking out.* Kansas City: Andrews McMeel Publishing.
Worell, J., & Johnson, N.G. (Eds.) (1997). *Shaping the future of feminist psychology.*
    Washington, DC: American Psychological Association.

From Life-Threatening Illness
to a More Sensitive Therapist:
One Woman's Journey

Juli Burnell

SUMMARY. This article describes the author's connection between a life-threatening illness and the personal and professional transformation she underwent. In particular, it discusses the impact on sense of self, the value of collaboration, the use of self-disclosure, and the importance of systemic sensitivity in the therapeutic process. *[Article copies available for a fee from The Haworth Document Delivery Service: 1-800-342-9678. E-mail address: <getinfo@haworthpressinc.com> Website: <http://www.HaworthPress.com> ©2001 by The Haworth Press, Inc. All rights reserved.]*

KEYWORDS. Illness, feminist therapy, self, collaboration, self-disclosure

Juli Burnell, PsyD, is a psychologist and Coordinator of Groups and Workshops in the Counseling Center at the University of Dayton.

The author wishes to thank Melinda Murphy, RMT, Nicole Thomas, LMT, and Mary Jo Rugierri, PhD, RPP, for their ongoing collaboration in her healing process; Kerry Glaus, PhD, PsyD, and Ellyn Kaschak, PhD, for help with revisions; and Gail Krumheuer, BS, for her editorial assistance. Special thanks go to Cindy Shaw, MS, PC, a fellow traveler in the challenge of chronic illness, for continued support of personal and professional endeavors.

Address correspondence to: Juli Burnell, University of Dayton Counseling Center, 300 College Park, Dayton, OH 45469-0910 (E-mail: juli.burnell@notes.udayton.edu).

[Haworth co-indexing entry note]: "From Life-Threatening Illness to a More Sensitive Therapist: One Woman's Journey." Burnell, Juli. Co-published simultaneously in *Women & Therapy* (The Haworth Press, Inc.) Vol. 23, No. 1, 2001, pp. 121-130; and: *Minding the Body: Psychotherapy in Cases of Chronic and Life-Threatening Illness* (ed: Ellyn Kaschak) The Haworth Press, Inc., 2001, pp. 121-130. Single or multiple copies of this article are available for a fee from The Haworth Document Delivery Service [1-800-342-9678, 9:00 a.m. - 5:00 p.m. (EST). E-mail address: getinfo@haworthpressinc.com].

The irony of nearly dying is that, for many people, it is a life-giving event. So it has been for me. Someone once said to me, "Serenity is not freedom from the storm but peace within the storm." In this article, I would like to describe my process of getting to the peace within the storm and the ways in which that process has informed my beliefs and practice of psychotherapy.

THE STORM

Approximately four years ago, just two days after my return from having presented a paper at The Association for Women in Psychology (AWP) Conference in Portland, Oregon, I awoke to an excruciating headache, double vision, and an inability to balance my body. After being taken to physicians of several different specialties that day, none of whom could diagnose my condition, I ended up in the emergency room undergoing an MRI. It was determined that I suffered from an abscess in the right side of my brainstem—the area that controls breathing, consciousness, and through which run nerves that orchestrate movement and enable vision. I was rushed to the Intensive Care Unit and was started on a course of round-the-clock intravenous antibiotics in the hope that the origin of the abscess was bacterial, and that "they could kill it before it killed me." Within forty-eight hours, I had suffered left-sided paralysis and was intermittently losing consciousness. At that point, the surgery against which the neurosurgeon had strongly recommended just twenty-four hours earlier because of the high risk of permanent paralysis, blindness, or death, was undertaken in an attempt to relieve the pressure in my brain and to culture the agent of the infection.

During the four weeks that followed, I felt like a prisoner in a nightmare that I believed would never end. Nurses woke me every two hours to change IV bags. The antibiotics burned through almost every IV site on the top half of my body. Once I learned about and insisted upon the insertion of a permanent IV receptacle, this central line was installed in my right arm. Almost every time I tried to move, the line would plug up, the IV apparatus would begin to beep, and after several minutes a nurse would arrive to reset it and give me a scolding for occluding the line.

Since it often took many minutes to obtain nursing assistance, and since I couldn't stand up without help, I was in constant fear of needing bathroom assistance. I therefore limited my water intake even though I knew that to do so was putting my liver at risk due to the toxicity of the antibiotics. The physicians were upset with me for voicing despair about my continuing inability to move or see after the abscess was under control. They couldn't understand why their former promises that I'd be back to normal once the abscess was healing had contributed to my sense of hopelessness. The neurosurgeon's response was, "It's a miracle that you're alive. That should be enough." In addition, I had just given the workshop at AWP, where I talked at length about how we create our reality. Unfortunately, I was now simplifying this to mean that improper beliefs had caused my illness and that if I believed hard enough, I should be able instantly to "fix" myself. These experiences compounded my sense of lack of control to the point where I became suicidal. For the first time in my life, I felt that my emotional pain and perceived loss of self were so great that death seemed like a comfort. Or at least death would be a way for me to reclaim control by stopping the loss and pain.

I spent two and a half weeks in intensive care, ten days in inpatient rehabilitation, and four months in outpatient rehabilitation where I learned to walk again, to see with double vision only at the periphery, to move my left side and to function independently–with the only vestige a tremor of intension in my left hand so that, for example, tying my shoes is a challenge. It remains unknown how I contracted the intestinal streptococcus bacteria that caused the abscess, how the bacteria got into my brain, or if it could happen again.

My self-concept before the storm was built on my athleticism, my quickness of thought, my independence, and my ability to overcome anything that stood in my way. As I lay in the hospital, I couldn't understand why friends kept coming to visit. After all, I couldn't "do" anything for them, not even be entertaining. The one person who directly experienced more of my vulnerability, my partner, was unprepared for this change in me. She became understandably upset by my pleas to gain her assistance in ending my life. Each morning seemed unbearable as I realized I had ahead of me another day of pain and frustration, combined with a lack of potential for self-determination or life satisfaction. I relived the terror that I had felt in childhood when my depressed mother was often unresponsive and treated my needs as a source of threat. This was compounded by my partner's withdrawal. She came to see me for increasingly shorter periods and vowed to stop coming altogether if I didn't stop talking about suicide. She reinforced my beliefs that I was creating my own reality, stating that maybe I had brought on this illness in some way to impact our relationship. Looking back, I surmise that she was limited in her availability to me due to her background from an enmeshed family system in which she was called to meet adults' needs. She never got beyond the initial fear of accepting my helplessness. So even when I came home with a fairly positive attitude and without the need of a great deal of physical assistance, she continued to see me as "too needy" and left the relationship two months later. I felt intense grief at my losses of health, self-concept, independence, and love, which included the death of my beloved fifteen-year-old cat while I was in the hospital, and the departure of my partner after I came home.

Five months after this "storm," I returned to my work as a psychologist in the Counseling Center at the University of Dayton. I have given you this much detail about my experience because my therapeutic beliefs and practices have changed and strengthened as a result of this experience.

GETTING THE PEACE

Once home, I began to see how healing is not an all-or-nothing proposition. As time went on, I became acutely aware of the ways in which long-term, chronic illness was changing my perception of myself. I also realized that I had to establish ongoing self-care practices to deal with my grief. Within this realization came an effort to move away from the myth that if I tried hard enough I could overcome anything. I incorporated Harold Kushner's (1983) ideas about letting go of the illusion that if this bad thing happened, I must have caused or deserved it. I read Susan Sontag's (1978) thoughts on the metaphorical thinking and corresponding stigmatization of illness as weakness. I embraced the idea that responsibility means not blaming anyone or anything for my situation, including myself.

I learned much about focusing, or rather *not just* focusing, on symptoms. It was difficult not to be so outcome-oriented as to focus only on being able to walk or being able to carry a glass of water with my left hand. However, focusing only on "being all better" didn't provide me much hope, since the symptoms were present for a long time and, in the case of my hand, still are. When I focused only on the symptoms, my experience was failure and despair. Then one day, when I was able to move the thumb on my left hand for the first time in months, it seemed so amazing to me. How was it possible that one day I thought, "Move" and nothing happened, and the next I thought "Move" and it did? That was the point at which I began focusing on the process. I became empowered. Yes, I still grieved over the necessary redefinition of myself. But now, I could also begin to see improvements in who I was as a result of this process. Now I could begin to claim my worth as a person and not for what I did. I learned that I had value just for being in other's lives. I learned that my life had value for the sheer sake of learning about and growing into myself. I was now free creatively to respond to my life as it was in each moment.

WORKING FROM THE PEACE

As I grew into the peace and into belief of my own inherent value as an experiential being, my view of myself as a therapist also grew. I was surprised and dismayed as I looked back on past work through the lens of having been on the other side of a healing relationship. Some of my former practices and beliefs probably had the opposite result of what I had intended. Though I had always believed in feminist principles, through the process of my illness I was able to see how I still carried some vestiges of beliefs that I was responsible for my clients' welfare, that I should control certain of their behaviors, and that at times I needed to be the expert. The impact of my own ordeal both personally and professionally was to stop me from taking anything for granted, to appreciate each moment, and to be more mindful about the "shoulds" that I follow. I believe that, in particular, this near-death experience has greatly increased my empathy for my clients' struggles. It has more acutely focused my use of feminist principles. As a framework for discussing my learnings about principles, I organize them below as Worell and Remer (1992) have previously as *"Egalitarian Relationships, Valuing the Female Perspective* and the *Personal Is Political"* (p. 91).

The first principle of which I became acutely aware was the importance of the establishment of an *Egalitarian Relationship* (Rosewater & Walker, 1985; Howard, 1986). My greatest emotional struggles during my hospitalization and beyond came from the loss of the control that I felt at having been "done to" without my input. I had always worked from the belief that my clients and I were partners in our therapeutic endeavors. Or so I thought. Then I began to explore my practices with clients who self-mutilate or with bulimics who are referred by our residential program staff. I realized that, in a fashion similar to the systematically forced IV treatments, I would impose the writing of logs and performing of certain prescribed behavioral steps. It is not that these tools aren't useful or that, just as in my case, the situation doesn't sometimes call for life-saving intervention. But the process of coming to the intervention does make all the difference. For example, I set a clear boundary that I cannot work effectively with a client who continually engages in self-mutilation. I no longer believe that she has to stop or that it is up to me to stop her. With eating disordered clients, our Counseling Center staff now uses a protocol that provides a structured way for clients to assess their current levels of functioning and motivation for change. They can focus their work in the areas of body image, eating behavior, wellness, and self-esteem. They can also decide honestly that they are not ready to change anything. We give clients a statement of our philosophy that says that we will support them in working on what they choose to do, and that it is fine not to do everything now.

Both of these examples respect the clients' and my own rates of development. Through my illness experience, I moved from a rather undiscerned ideal of myself and the client as equals to a more sophisticated belief about our relationship as egalitarian. As Brown (1994) says, " . . . a primary goal is for the client to come to value her own needs and knowledge as central . . . the

therapist is present . . . to resonate with, mirror, and engage the client . . . "
(p. 104). Thinking back, it would have made such a difference if hospital
personnel had worked with me by setting the parameters, e.g., you must have
an IV change every two hours, but then requesting my input about things like
the IV site and how that impacted my physical therapy. After having been
subjected to a delivery system that is set up to disempower patients, I work
harder not to recreate that in my clinical setting.

The second tenet, *Valuing the Female Perspective,* applies on several
different levels. Feminist therapists work within community (Greenspan,
1983). Also, as Worell and Remer (1992) remind us, it is important to revalue
traditional female characteristics such as cooperation, intuition, and interdependence. I therefore now often work within a community of healers by
recommending collaboration with alternative practitioners. Utilizing professionals from outside the mainstream medical model enhances a focus on
collaboration and process rather than simply on outcome. I have seen how a
team effort with a polarity therapist, massage therapist, Alexander movement
therapist, herbalist, aromatherapist, and acupuncturist have deepened, en-
riched, and accelerated my own therapy and healing. For example, as I
continue to work toward normal functioning of my left hand, my experiences
with my Alexander teacher remind me of several key principles over and
over again (Conable, 1997). I am still often drawn to focus on my hand when
it trembles; it is only after seeing the tremor reduction that results from doing
exercises to lengthen my spine and encourage arm, shoulder, and torso syn-
chronicity that I recall lessons about focusing on the process instead of the
symptom. This movement work also reminds me that sometimes less is more.
That is, as I stop trying to force the movement and instead focus on the
process by performing at a level that is currently achievable, I obtain a better
outcome. Clients who are "survivors" are often amazed that learning to care
for their inner children is more successful than constantly focusing on symptoms that were a result of their abuse. This is parallel to my experience in that
attending to the whole person and encouraging the client to move away from
an attempt to fix symptoms is transformative.

In consultation with a Polarity therapist, I have seen that working with my
energy system is helpful in exploring conditioned responses. Polarity therapy
(Sills, 1991) is an excellent complement to my work with clients because it
addresses the interdependence of body, mind, and spirit, the importance of
relationships, and the value of creating a way of balance in life. A basic tenet
of Polarity Therapy, as of Feminist Therapy, is that the client already knows
but has lost touch with what needs to happen within her body/heart/mind to
heal. Through these different mediums, we can work collaboratively to help
restore balance.

All of these forms of collaborative alternative medicine require input from the client and focus on the process for them even to be undertaken. My therapeutic endeavors are so much more effective when both the client and I can see how therapy is a process. Even though the symptom of paralysis made it appear that I wasn't improving, the process of change was occurring. Based on my experience, a collaborative team approach that combines body workers, energy workers, and psychotherapists assists all to focus more on the process of our own inner knowing and the power of the relationships among us. In this way, the team and the client attend more to how the client is growing, rather than simply to symptom relief.

As I focus on the process from an egalitarian, collaborative frame, I am now much more effective in my use of self-disclosure. My self-disclosures help to balance the power between myself and my clients while encouraging them to focus on both the intrapsychic and the external social conditions we share. By telling them of our similar experiences, I can model valuing of the female experience as well as provide a deeper level of empathy. My personal experience has changed the amount and timing of my self-disclosures, as well as the types of clients to whom I disclose.

For example, prior to my own illness it was only theory that caused me to explore the possibility that a client's suicidal ideation might be a final effort to gain some control. Before, I had no personal frame of reference from which to understand the depths of despair that leave some clients with the inability to imagine improvement. I have found it extremely powerful in sparking hope to be able to share my own experiences. It is helpful for clients to hear about the steps I went through beyond the initial sense of hopelessness: my initial surprise that I could get through the despair, my physical and emotional improvement, and my gratitude now that I am alive. Saying that things often do get better no longer seems discounting. Several of my clients have reported that hearing parts of my experience was a turning point toward becoming aware of more possibilities.

Similarly, I now have a different understanding of, and can more effectively communicate, the terror that sometimes accompanies a regressive experience. Had I understood all the aspects of my terror when I was in the hospital, I think it would have made it more manageable. When I self-disclose parts of my regression experiences to clients, they often report feeling more normal and more able to withstand their own encounters with it. For example, when abuse survivors become "little and scared" in my office, I can help to provide a container and can be an anchor for them. I can help them to make sense of the process.

As I become more astute at intervening according to the third feminist principle, the *Personal Is Political,* I pay much more attention to the benefits of working within a client's personal and societal social systems. This way I can help them to understand the ways that stereotyping and oppression within these systems limit their potential and contribute to their pain. In past work, I discussed with clients possible ramifications of change on their social system. I helped clients explore the impact that personal, peer, and societal messages were having on them. After having had the experiences of being ignored or spoken to as if I were retarded because I was in a wheelchair; after having been surprised by my partner's leaving the relationship when I was steadily improving, I became more convinced of the need to focus on societal messages and to intervene earlier with a client's support network. I was told by the rehabilitation team that worked with me that the most typical responses to change by clients' support systems are to leave or to subvert change to maintain homeostasis. I incorporate this knowledge into my assessment of clients' systems.

In my work at a university, I have seen ways in which the external systems are the main source of clients' problems. Thus the primary sources of many client difficulties are social and political, not simply personal and intrapsychic. An obvious and frequently seen example of societal level impact on a college campus is the Euro-American, male student who realizes he is getting into dangerous territory with alcohol and decides to cut back or stop drinking. The constant barrage of messages from television sitcoms and commercials, as well as campus paraphernalia that mostly references drinking, all attest to the necessity of alcohol for having a good time and being a "real (dominant culture) man." So the student gets reminded at every turn that he is being "weird" by not drinking. Then of course there's the reaction of his social network. His partner, who may have even previously voiced concern about his level of alcohol consumption, starts complaining that the couple is becoming isolated or that the client is "no fun anymore." Buddies stop asking the client to "hang out" with them. So I help the client to prepare for these reactions by examining his own and his social network's beliefs about masculinity and drinking. This lessens the societal impact on the client and hopefully prevents his return to old patterns of usage and subsequent disappearance from treatment.

An example of systemic impact at the cultural and familial levels can be seen by examining the work a Latina client and I did to help her to set limits with her family. She was going home every weekend to care for her grandmother, so that the remainder of the family could rest on weekends. As a result, she had no study time on weekends and was often too exhausted to attend class during the week. She said that she felt caught between the expectations of her traditional Mexican-American family and those of her liberal Euro-American college peers. Vasquez (1994) talks about the importance of the family in Chicano culture, about how the individuation process is different for clients from that culture, and that the Chicana's emphasis on familial responsibilities is often related to academic difficulties. Therefore, while the client presented stating that she needed to learn to meet all of the demands within her social system, in therapy she was able to identify the impact of these conflicting demands. I validated the nurturing skills she already utilized with her family and helped her to learn how to apply those to herself as well. She began voicing to her family that she still loved them even when she needed to set limits with them in order to be loving with herself. She developed the ability to examine potential consequences and then to make choices that were supportive of herself within her familial and peer social contexts. The exploration of external factors as causative in clients' problems is a powerful intersection of both feminist and cross-cultural therapy principles.

The importance of an understanding of external factors can be seen at the systemic level of the couple as well. This was evident in a discussion I recently had with a supervisee concerning an abused Euro-American female client. She was pleased to have helped the client to set some limits with an abusive boyfriend, but was struggling to accept the seemingly ironic increase in danger in which that stance put the client. She was struggling as well with the reaction of the client herself, who didn't like the loss of attention from her boyfriend that she experienced when he wasn't being abusive.

Therapists sometimes respond at the intrapsychic level to clients' confusion and pain by saying, "This is happening now because you are strong enough to handle it." When I was in the position of being a patient, I experienced this statement as very demoralizing. I now see this kind of statement as a variation of my simplified you-create-your-own-reality beliefs, the ones that didn't serve me well as I lay blaming myself for being paralyzed. I don't mean to imply that psychotherapy isn't hard work, that it doesn't have its ups and downs, or that things don't sometimes feel worse before they feel better. Not at all. Those are important things for the client to know about the process so that she can fully collaborate in it. But couldn't the above response be construed as encouraging self-blame as well? When I was first struggling to make sense of my illness, a friend suggested that I read *When Bad Things Happen to Good People* (Kushner, 1983). That book got me refocused toward looking at external cultural messages, instead of seeing the problem as simply within myself. Realizing that there is a cultural tenet that bad things *can't* happen to good people and that this tenet is a myth empowered me in ways similar to the ones I've described in the case examples above. Now, part of my work with all clients is to look carefully at self-talk and societal opinion, and to replace self-recrimination with self-affirmation.

It is quite a lesson for me to learn how struggling with a long-term illness has changed my self-concept. I have a different understanding of my clients who are living with clinical depression who say, "I just want to be who I used to be." The clients who do the best (myself included) are the ones who relinquish attempts to recapture the past and instead embrace all of who they are now. They are the ones who can experience growth from the illness process.

The impact of my illness experience on my work was eloquently described to me by a long-term graduate student client who had worked with me for a year prior to my illness and then again immediately following it. At a time when she felt in the depths of despair and uncertain as to whether she'd ever be able to change her body image/disordered eating behaviors, she said, "You know, sometimes I just don't want to go on. But after I talk to you, I feel like you really understand how hopeless I feel. And when I think about quitting, I think about how much you've gone through and how far you've come, and I figure if you were willing to keep trying, I can also." We are both growing from the processes involved in healing from our illnesses.

REFERENCES

Brown, L. S. (1994). *Subversive dialogues.* New York, NY: Basic Books.

Conable, B., & Conable, W. (1997). *How to learn the Alexander technique.* Columbus, OH: Andover Press.

Greenspan, M. (1983). *A new approach to women & therapy.* New York, NY: McGraw-Hill Book Company.

Howard, D. (Ed.). (1986). *The dynamics of feminist therapy.* New York, NY: The Haworth Press, Inc.

Kushner, H.S. (1983). *When bad things happen to good people.* New York, NY: Avon Books.

Rosewater, L. B., & Walker, L. E. A. (Eds.). (1985). *Handbook of feminist therapy: Women's issues in psychotherapy.* New York, NY: Springer Publishing Company.

Sills, F. (1991). *The polarity process.* Boston, MA: Element Books.

Sontag, S. (1978). *Illness as metaphor.* New York, NY: Doubleday.

Vasquez, M. J. T. (1994). Latinas. In L. Comas-Diaz & B. Greene (Eds.), *Women of color.* (pp. 114-138). New York, NY: The Guilford Press.

Worell, J., & Remer, P. (1992). *Feminist perspectives in therapy.* West Sussex, England: John Wiley & Sons Ltd.

Index

Accident, fibromyalgia exacerbation, account of, 60-61
ACR. *See* American College of Rheumatology
Activity level changes, body image and, 17
Acupuncture, illness and, 4
ADA. *See* Americans with Disabilities Act (ADA)
Adaptability, new constructs and, 92
Adjustment, chronic illness and, 8
Adjustment period, tasks of, 11-12
Advocacy, therapist and, 53
Air quality
    research needed, 34
    in sealed buildings, 27-29
    symptoms from toxic, 27-29
Air quality standards, Ontario, 31
Allergies
    Sick Building Syndrome and, 32
    symptom of Chronic Fatigue Syndrome, 24
    allopathic medicine, medicine as science metaphor and, 77-78
ALS, distinguished from fibromyalgia, 49
American College of Rheumatology
    criteria for classification of fibromyalgia, 48-49
    fibromyalgia syndrome and, 46
American Medical Association, Sick Building Syndrome and, 39
Americans with Disabilities Act (ADA)
    accommodations required under, 73
    employment discrimination despite, 82-83
Anger
    at arrogance of neurosurgeon, first-hand account (of Denise Twohey), 118

at chronic illness, 53
as a means of coping, 82
Anger management techniques, feminist therapists and, 18
Anxiety
    autoimmune disorders and, 11
    breast cancer and, 104
        first-hand account, 104
    chronic illness and, 8
    fibromyalgia and, 50-51
Anxiety management techniques, feminist therapists and, 18
Assertiveness training, feminist therapists and, 18
Association for Women in Psychology (AWP), 122,123
Athletic pursuits, change of sport needed, 17
Attitude, cancer survival and, 83
Autoimmune diseases. *See also* Autoimmune disorders
    reality of, 3
Autoimmune disorders
    acknowledgment of avoided by healthy individuals, 16
    age of onset, 9
    autoantibodies and, 9
    cancer and, 1
    characteristics of, 7
    common, 9
    course of, 10-11
    endocrine functioning alteration and, 10
    environmental factors contributing to, 10
    experience with, 7,10-11
    genetic factors contributing to, 10
    incidence of, 7
        gendered difference in, 9